BREAKTHROUGH DENTAL
MARKETING

BREAKTHROUGH DENTAL
MARKETING

A dentist's guide to getting
and keeping patients

JOEL HARRIS

aardvark
PUBLISHING

This book is dedicated to every dentist
who is ready to begin marketing.

Acknowledgments

This book has been written from many years of experience working with everything from the world's largest corporations to the smallest businesses. These entities all share the same need to effectively market themselves to the world. It has been fascinating to study and learn from each of them. Every business makes mistakes and a few of them have incredible successes. Hopefully, I've picked up a few things a long the way that I can pass along.

I would like to thank every partner and associate I've had along the way. I've learned something from all of them.

I'd like to thank my wife Janice for putting up with me while I wrote this book. She was a great support and helped me stay focused and motivated while I finished this project.

I especially want to thank Dr. Robert Thorup for his never-ending confidence and positive attitude. It is my hope that we'll continue to work together for a long time.

Finally, I want to acknowledge the brilliant team of experts at Intelligent Dental Marketing for their commitment to help dental professionals grow, profit, and thrive.

Contents

Introduction

The idea for Breakthrough Marketing came to me last year after finishing a small but information-packed little book about marketing small businesses. I love to read, and after years of assisting dental practices with marketing strategies and tactics, I decided that it was time to publish some ideas and thoughts that have had a profound impact on my success.

Every dentist needs to create and implement an effective marketing plan that is tailored for his or her community and type of practice. Over years, I have developed tools and systems that take the guess work out of this process. The results can be amazing. However, before these tools and systems can be utilized fully, the management team in a dental practice must begin to see the world differently. My partner calls it "putting on your business hat." That is where this book comes in.

As you read this book, I want you to see your practice just like every other small business owner sees his or her business. I want you to also try to see the world through the eyes of your patient. Put your instruments away, and open your mind to the ideas and business philosophies in this book. You will gain a new vision for what it is, that actually makes patients buy dental products and services. Most of all, I hope you enjoy the time you spend reading this book. It was fun to write it and I think it will be fun to read.

THE STARTING POINT

What is the Purpose of Marketing?

About ten years ago, I was in a seminar with one of the nation's most respected marketing gurus. He started his address by asking a few members of the audience what they believed the real purpose of marketing was. Each volunteer gave an answer that was insightful, but none could provide an answer that seemed to satisfy the speaker. Keep in mind that this audience was mostly made up of marketing professionals and advertising executives. As the answers kept on coming, the speaker continued to shake his head, indicating that nobody was getting close. After about a dozen pretty good answers this guru helped me understand marketing in a way that I will never forget. He simply said, "ladies and gentlemen, the purpose of marketing is to shorten the sales cycle."

Now, I know that most of you reading this book are from the dental industry, so let me help you translate the term "sales cycle" into dental terminology. "Sales cycle" is the process of a consumer scheduling an appointment and accepting treatment. These consumers include everyone from complete strangers who become new patients, to even the most loyal lifelong patients.

Shortening the sales cycle through marketing will simplify and improve so many other objectives within your practice. Marketing will smooth out your cash-flow bumps and facilitate treatment acceptance. Marketing will eliminate cancellations and improve patient referrals. But most of all, marketing will shorten the process of a total stranger becoming a loyal patient.

Never forget—the purpose of marketing is to shorten the sales cycle.

Like it or not, dentistry is a popularity contest

Some of us loved high school and some of us hated high school. The reasoning behind either opinion is that high school is really just one big popularity contest. For the popular students, life seemed to always be so easy. Teachers and coaches always gave popular students the benefit of the doubt. Other students flocked around the popular students and made them their heros. The popular students always seemed to have the secret formula for success and an endless source of confidence.

Dentistry, whether you like it or not is just like high school. Patients always migrate to dentists who are fun to be around and who "seem" to be successful. If you want to succeed in dentistry you've got to be popular.

Patients will naturally migrate to dentists who "seem" to be popular.

Get Some Help

The most important advice that I can give to a dentist, is to seek out a marketing expert and make that person an important part of their dental practice. Too many small business owners, including dentists are "do-it-yourselfers" and fail to get the most out of their businesses, because they don't retain the services of an experienced pro that has proven to be successful.

Imagine how ridiculous I would look if I decided to do my own dental work. What would you say to me if I was convinced that I could make my own crown at home and that you ought to charge me less than your full fee, because you were only going to have to prep the crown. I would just cement my own homemade crown myself with some epoxy I bought at Home Depot. Oh, and by the way, I think I need a root canal. Could you just send me home with some instructions so my wife and I can take care of it ourselves? I've got a small cordless drill and I'll find an endo file on e-Bay.

This may sound like an exaggeration, but unfortunately, it's not. A Marketing expert will save you time, money and pain. A seasoned marketing pro knows the art and science of marketing like you know dentistry.

Practice what you preach... hire a pro.

Marketing Indifference...
Your worst nightmare

Believe me when I say that one of the biggest problems facing dentistry today is the problem of marketing indifference. Nearly every business in the world relies heavily on marketing in one or more of its forms. Unfortunately, dental professionals from all over the country have been taught that marketing is either not necessary or doesn't work. I don't want to drive the analogy from the previous section into the ground, but not believing in marketing is like not believing in brushing your teeth. Maybe brushing is not all it's cracked up to be. Maybe if I just ignore all of that plaque on my teeth it'll just go away on its own.

Don't kid yourself – marketing works.

Analysis Paralysis

Quite frequently, I have the opportunity to teach dentists and their teams in a seminar setting. At a recent seminar, a dentist attended who had just added his recently graduated son as a new dentist in his practice. The plan was to bring in Junior, teach him the ropes and, in a few years, retire to Florida.

Unfortunately, the father found that sharing his patients with his son made it difficult to stay busy and profitable.

The other problem facing the dynamic duo, was a team of young and aggressive dentists across the street who were, as he put it, "stealing our patients with their slick advertising."

Due to his old-school philosophies, the father hated the idea of marketing his practice. He best described his position on marketing when he said, "I can't believe that dentistry has got to a point where I need to run an ad to get patients."

Out of fear, he spent months over-analyzing the situation. I know from conversations with him that his thoughts went something like this: What if it doesn't work? What will my peers think? Will we get too many patients? Should I get a second opinion? Maybe we should try something less expensive? And on and on.

Unfortunately, that father and son team continues to struggle. They have wasted month after month waiting for the perfect opportunity and the perfect time to begin marketing. Meanwhile, the dentists across the street continue to aggressively market their practice and thrive.

You'll never be able to afford the high cost of lost opportunity.

The parable of the wise fisherman

There once were two friends who were fisherman. For many years they had fished in the same part of the sea and had fed themselves and their families from the fish they caught and sold at market. Once, during a terrible storm, the two fisherman were separated and washed out to sea many miles away from shore, each in his own small boat. Neither fisherman had any extra food and very little water. However, each man had a few dead minnows that they used to bait their fishing lines. As each fisherman became more and more hungry they realized that catching fish to eat was the only way to survive the long journey back to the safety of land.

Both men tried without success to catch fish using their small ration of bait minnows. The first fisherman being very wise, realized that he must continue doing his best to catch a fish, so he carefully conserved his bait minnows until finally he was able to catch a fish on his last try with his last minnow. After eating his fill, this wise fisherman used part of the fish he caught for new bait and eventually caught several more fish. He was able to make it back to shore because of the energy he received from the fish he caught. He lived a long and prosperous life and learned not to go out to sea without being prepared for a storm.

The second fisherman was not a wise man and kept trying to catch fish with no success. When he saw that his bait minnows were dwindling he decided that the only choice he had was to eat the bait minnows he had left. He did not have the faith and wisdom of the wise fisherman and he eventually died of starvation while attempting to row his fishing boat back to land. His family never found his boat and they found it very difficult to provide for themselves for many years.

I wrote this little parable to help explain in simple terms how important it is to invest your "bait" or money into marketing your dental practice. If executed properly, it will bring you a much greater return for years to come. Don't ignore this wisdom. Don't wait until it is too late and don't be tempted to eat your bait.

Eating your bait will result in the same outcome every time –No more bait.

DENTAL MARKETING
FALLACIES

Marketing is unethical

For reasons that are completely foreign to me, the dental community still harbors negative opinions about any kind of external marketing or advertising. I know that a lot of this negativity stems from old-school dentists who were fortunate to practice during a time when simply being a dentist guaranteed a certain amount of success. I've spoken with dentists who, in years past, were even shunned by their peers for running a simple newspaper ad. The philosophy being perpetuated, was that these renegade dentists were going to somehow taint the whole industry and turn dentists into ambulance-chasers or used-car salesmen.

Fortunately, times are changing. We live in a world where marketing is a vital part of the success of any business. Advertising agencies, technology advancements and the media in general have created an intense, fast-paced world where name brands, discount clubs and multi-million dollar advertising campaigns rule the world. Dental professionals who fail to recognize and understand the rules of this ever-changing game, will struggle to thrive in the new century.

Believing it is unethical for dentists to market their practices can be a dangerous assumption.

Marketing makes me look desperate

The largest companies in the world, spend billions of dollars on complex marketing campaigns, because they know that being the biggest and the best today may change tomorrow. The leaders of these mega corporations are far from desperate. They're not begging for business and they don't apologize for pitching their products and services.

Dentists who intelligently market their practices are not desperate. They are shrewd business people who understand the necessity of creating continual awareness for their products and services.

Market your practice now. You won't look desperate, you'll look smart.

I didn't go to dental school to be a salesman

I either hear this phrase word for word, or I see it in the eyes of too many dentists. In one form or another, I have been a salesman all of my life. I don't wear a plaid sport coat and I don't use tacky sales pitches. I am proud to be a good salesman and have found success in my life because of it. Some of the most influential people in the world are some of the world's best salespeople. Steve Jobs didn't build Apple Computer because he's a talented nerd. He built Microsoft because he is a brilliant salesman and marketing genius. Sam Walton, the founder of Wal-Mart, Walt Disney, Henry Ford, Thomas Edison and the other great founders of business empires were all great salespeople. They weren't famous for being pushy. They were famous for being able to sell.

All of the successful dentists I have met over the years are all very accomplished salespeople. They didn't build thriving practices behind a mask with their hands in a patient's mouth. They built their practices because they learned how to communicate with their patients. They learned how to build relationships and they learned how to get their patients to say "yes"—all talents of a good salesperson.

Don't despise selling—become good at it.

I'll do my marketing on trade

Please don't make the mistake of doing your marketing on trade! It happens all too often and the results are almost always the same. The dentist does several thousand dollars of dental work and the graphic design and marketing work never quite gets finished. Usually, the quality is average at best and your patient doesn't know a crown from a filling. I've seen it so many times, I've lost count.

Patients who can't afford dentistry probably aren't the best source of marketing expertise. Trade for carpet cleaning or credit at the hardware store. Never trade for dental marketing services. Find a professional and be willing to pay them.

Remember, you get what you pay for.

I can't afford a professional

A good dental marketing professional is worth every penny. When a marketing plan is properly executed it won't cost you anything. It will only make money. I tell dentists every day that marketing doesn't have to be seen as a long-term investment. It works quickly and in many cases the return is so rapid, that the initial expense of the campaign is back in the bank within the first few weeks.

Hiring an experienced professional can get you these kinds of results. When you need legal help, hire an attorney. When you need accounting help hire an accountant. When you need marketing help, hire a pro.

You can't afford not to hire a professional.

When I need patients, I'll start marketing

Marketing should be seen as preventative medicine not just a cure for your problem. Wise dentists, like all wise business owners, are always marketing. They don't wait until the well is dry to solve the problem.

Even if you think you've got plenty of patients, the attrition rate of the average dental practice is high enough to warrant a consistent and perpetual marketing plan. I don't know a dentist who couldn't use some help replacing lost patients who have had to change dentists because they either moved, divorced, changed insurance, or a host of other issues.

Marketing isn't a thing you do every so often, it should be a way of life.

I have plenty of patients

I need to be very careful how I explain my philosophy with regard to this section, so here goes. Unless a patient is in your office he or she is not yours. Any patient that is not on their back with their mouth open in your chair may have already started seeing another dentist for reasons you may never know.

I have always found it cavalier when a dentist gives me their official "patient count." I am especially suspect of these head counts, because I am in the business of helping dentists grow their practices. Quite often, the new patients we help dentists attract, respond to an offer or an ad because they are at some level not satisfied with their current dentist.

In almost every practice, there is a core of active patients that make up the bulk of the business. Take care of these patients like gold, because they are. In addition, there are a multitude of potential patients who are looking for a dentist due to a number of factors. Some studies state that 25% of all persons 18 years of age and over haven't seen a dentist in over 2 years! Now, be willing to admit that a patient who hasn't been in your office in two years, may very well be visiting another dentist and somewhere along the way you lost that patient's loyalty. It doesn't mean you are a bad dentist, it only goes to show you that some other dentist out-marketed you. It may have been through something as subtle as location, or as aggressive as a free offer from a new kid on the block. Either way you lost, and to ensure that it doesn't affect your profitability next time, make sure you implement your own marketing plan to attract those consumers who are in the market for a dentist.

Think twice next time you count your patients.

WHAT DO PATIENTS REALLY WANT?

Patients assume you sterilize

As I travel around the country, I frequently take the time to open the yellow pages in my hotel room to check out the local dental marketing climate. Unfortunately, it is always the same. Dentist after dentist, making the same claims and benefits that mean nothing to the average patient. The most over-used claim is "Dr. Jones uses modern sterilization equipment to protect your health." The problem with such a claim, is that patients already assume that dentists sterilize their equipment. It's like assuming that a restaurant washes their dishes.

In addition to the sterilization line there are plenty of other lackluster claims. "Comprehensive Dentistry", "Now Accepting New Patients", "Quality Care" and the list goes on and on.

Only dentists know what comprehensive dentistry really means, and patients assume you are accepting new patients or you wouldn't be running an ad.

Make your advertising count for something. Differentiate your message. Get creative.

Appeal to their emotions

Promote your practice in a way that appeals to a person's emotions. Sell the public the emotional advantage of using your services. Tell them how beautiful they will look. Profile before and after photography everywhere. Don't hide your new equipment behind closed doors. Sell your patients on the cutting edge equipment you use and how it will make their life better. Explain very simply, how easy it is to pay and how nobody waits in your reception area for more than a few moments. Use color, use photos.

Consumers have emotional hot buttons. Find them and push them whenever you can.

Don't be the best, be good enough

An important piece of advice I would give to any dentist is; *don't be too good*. This may seem like strange advice from someone who is supposed to help you improve your practice, so let me explain.

I meet a lot of dentists. As scientists and medical experts, they were all taught to research, study, analyze and methodically make decisions. By nature, many of them struggle with needing to be perfect in all areas of their professional life. As a result, they often over-analyze and over-think. It's called analysis paralysis. It's the sickness of not doing anything for fear of making a mistake. I see too many dentists who don't market themselves for fear of not being ready.

Now, don't get me wrong. We should all appreciate the fact that as medical professionals dentists are methodical and make every attempt to be clinically sound. However, my observation is that when dentists let this scientific philosophy govern the way they run their businesses, profitability and practice growth suffer.

Some dentists wait for the perfect plan to present itself. Sometimes, they wait for the perfect facility or the perfect team. Sometimes, they wait for the perfect equipment or the perfect material before they feel ready to market their practice. In the mean time, patients are scheduling appointments somewhere else.

What patients really want is a good dentist, that seems friendly has a fairly professional facility, and a nice team of people. Patients, like all consumers, don't usually make the best choice, they make the safest choice. In fact, most patients don't really know how to judge one dentist from another. Patients don't know the difference between an expensive filling material and a cheap one. Patients don't know how to look for a short margin on a crown. Patients are more concerned with the superficial things, like your reception area, and did your office manager remember their name. Most of the time, patients just don't want to make a bad choice.

Remember, perfection is the enemy of good enough.

People hate to go to the dentist... eliminate their fear

Anything you can do in your practice to eliminate the "fear factor" should be a priority. People, for the most part, hate pain. That's no mystery, but dental practices get way too comfortable with pain. The sound of the drill, the long needles, and the white knuckles are all in a day's work. A pain-free procedure is a great investment in the patient experience bank. Many dentists now offer sleep dentistry and conscious sedation options for their patients. In fact, if properly presented, these sedation options can create an important and unique selling point. I know a dentist who gives his patient the option to "fly first class, business or coach." First class is a sedation tablet. Business Class is Nitrous Oxide. And, coach is Novocaine. His patients love the option to decide how comfortable they want to be, and the more comfortable the patient, the more loyal they will be, which in-turn will increase profits.

Fear Factor is a great reality show. It's a bad reputation for your dental practice.

Above all, sell hope

More important than anything else, instill a feeling of hope in the lives of your patients. Many people have never maintained their teeth like they should have because they have lost hope of ever having a great smile. They feel like it is too late. Maybe they've smoked for years or had terribly crooked teeth. Maybe they were told one too many times when they were growing up, that they didn't fit in. Maybe they were raised in a home where dental care was never important because it was too expensive. Maybe they've dreamed of having a great smile, but they haven't had a whole lot to smile about.

That's where an extraordinary dentist is different from a pretty good dentist. Giving your patients the ability to smile again is a wonderful gift. Make the most out of it. I've seen lives completely altered for the better because a patient finally learned how to smile at the world without being embarrassed or self-conscious. No, not every patient can have a Hollywood smile, but every patient can be given a chance to hope again. It may take awhile to make practice-wide changes and this philosophy might not be right for everyone on your dental team. If you have a team member who won't make a commitment to sell hope, make a change right away and find someone who can.

Learn to see the world through the eyes of every individual patient and give the gift of hope.

WHAT DO YOUR PATIENTS REALLY THINK?

They'll lie to your face...

I frequently talk to office managers, who tell me that "patients just love our practice" or "Everybody loves Dr. Jones." I don't buy it. I'm not saying that some patients don't love Dr. Jones but more often than not, if a patient has a bad experience, Dr. Jones and his team will never know about it.

The problem dentists face, is that their patients will rarely tell them how they actually feel. Now, I know that every office has had experiences with the occasional outspoken patient but for the most part, patients quietly bite their lip while they're in the office and then rush home and tell their friends and family why they'll never go to that dentist again!

Next time you hear that you are loved by everyone—take it with a grain of salt.

...But they'll spill their guts to a stranger

I f you really want to know how you are doing and how your patients really feel about your practice, you need to hire an independent company to conduct a survey. It won't cost a lot and can be accomplished in a few days.

Usually a random sampling of 50 to 100 patients will tell you everything you need to know.

Companies who serve the public have relied on independent surveys for years because they work. Entire firms have been built to do nothing but get feedback from consumers. Most of the time when you purchase a new car, you will receive a phone call within a few days from an independent caller. This caller's job is to find out how you *really* felt about your buying experience. Most of us are more than willing to be completely honest because there is no pressure to fake it. I know that if the salesman himself called, most of us would give a totally different answer.

Responses to questions should be kept anonymous to make the respondent completely comfortable with being honest. The survey questions should really get to the point and should go something like this: "Are Dr. Jones and his team as concerned about you as they should be"? "If you could improve anything at Dr. Jones practice, what would it be"?   "Have you ever considered using another dentist"? and so on.

Sometimes reality can be a bitter pill to take, and other times it can be a reassuring validation of hard work and effort. Either way, don't fall into the fallacy that ignorance is bliss.

If you really want to know how you are doing, hire an independent firm to find out.

MARKETING STRATEGY
VS.
MARKETING TACTICS

Strategy vs. tactics

Every business owner needs to understand the difference between a marketing strategy and a marketing tactic. Having a well-defined strategy and employing effective tactics, is an age-old rule that applies to successful warfare, political races, scientific discovery, athletic achievement and empire building.

When a military general decides to take a hill or beach-head because of the dominant position that will be achieved, a strategy has been created. It is a global plan, and the guiding purpose behind a series of smaller tasks.

The step-by-step assignments and jobs related to a mission or plan are tactics. Military operations can fail because a strategy is weak even though the tactics are executed flawlessly. The opposite is also true. A brilliant strategy may flop because the tactical planning and execution of critical tasks fail.

The right strategy and well executed tactics are both critical to any dental marketing effort. Too many dentists have a few great tactics with no long-term plan or objective. Other dentists may have the vision and the ideal strategy, without the resources or discipline to deploy the all-important marketing tactics.

There is a big difference between creating a marketing strategy and deploying marketing tactics

Most dentists don't have a strategy

U nfortunately, like most small business owners, dentists rarely have an overall strategy. If I asked most dentists, they would say that their strategy is to see a lot of patients and make a good living. This isn't a strategy! A strategy is a guiding focus. A strategy is a goal. A strategy is a vision.

Good examples of dental marketing strategies are:

Double the size of my patient base in 12 months.

Increase my profitability by 20 percent.

Open two new practices over five years.

Become recognized as a top implant dentist.

SOME PRINCIPLES
OF MARKETING

The cold hard facts

Take any 100 men or women at the start of their working careers, and follow them for 40 years till they reach retirement age. Here's what the Social Security Administration says you'll find:

- One will be wealthy.
- Four will be financially secure.
- Five will continue working because they have to.
- 36 will be dead.
- 54 will be broke—dependent on Social Security checks.

Hopefully, understanding these marketing principles will make you part of the 5%, not the 95% who struggle.

It's scary, but it's reality.

Keep it simple stupid

Most of the population, even business executives, do not understand the basic structure of marketing, and what tactics and disciplines are sub-categories of what I call the "Marketing Umbrella."

As I discussed in the first chapter, the purpose of marketing is to shorten the sales cycle. advertising, branding, public relations and customer service are all parts of the marketing family. Also, understand that

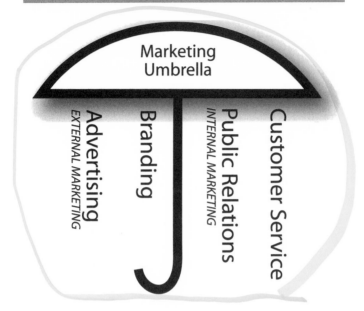

Marketing Umbrella

Advertising — EXTERNAL MARKETING

Branding

Public Relations — INTERNAL MARKETING

Customer Service

many, sub-categories or disciplines can fall under the umbrella of marketing. For more complex strategies, other sub-categories may include: polling, demography, packaging, copy writing, market research, and on and on. For a dental practice these are over-the-top so don't freak out. I won't mention them again. For the purposes of this book I have kept the list of marketing sub-categories to four. They are illustrated above, and as I've said, they all lead to sales. Or, for dentists... Case Acceptance.

Another misconception, is believing that marketing and advertising are the same thing. Or, that marketing

is another word to describe selling. For the purpose of
this book, you will see advertising and public relations
sometimes described as external and internal marketing.

Marketing isn't advertising and it isn't selling.
It's much, much more.

Frequency or reach?

R each is the number of people you touch with your
marketing message or the number of people that
are exposed to your message. Frequency is the number
of times you touch each person with your message. In
a world of unlimited resources you would obviously
maximize both reach and frequency. However, since
most of us live in the world of limited resources we must
often make decisions to sacrifice reach for frequency or
vice versa. In the case of a dental practice, money can be
wasted on marketing strategies that have too much reach
because of travel limitations of prospective patients.

A dental practice in Anaheim, California that has decided
to do a direct mail piece has to decide whether to mail
the entire Orange County area once or to mail a much
smaller area surrounding the practice many times.
Another dentist who likes the idea of running a radio ad
in Dallas, Texas will need to decide if it a wise decision to
run an ad that many thousands of people will hear, that

may live more than 50 miles from the practice.

When faced with decisions of reach vs. frequency remember this rule of thumb: Reach without frequency = wasted marketing money. Have you ever established a lifelong friendship with someone you had contact with only once? Probably not. Generally, friendships (and all relationships for that matter) grow as a result of frequent contact over time. Even when the potential to form a great friendship is there at the first encounter, it is unlikely it will grow without nurturing.

Seth Godin, in his book Permission Marketing, uses an analogy of seeds and water to demonstrate the importance of assuring adequate frequency in your promotional campaigns. If you were given 100 seeds with enough water to water each seed once would you plant all 100 seeds and water each one just one time. Or, would you be more successful if you planted 25 seeds and used all of the water on those 25 seeds?

Even though most dentists conceptually understand the importance of frequency to ensure a successful marketing campaign, somehow when it comes to actually implementing the plan, too many opt to choose reach over frequency. And then complain about the ineffectiveness of their marketing efforts. Sometimes, the idea of hearing their ad on the radio or seeing a gigantic billboard on a major freeway is just too hard to turn down. Unfortunately, it's usually a hard lesson to learn.

When faced with the decision of mailing one direct mail piece to 50,000 people, or mailing to 5,000 people ten times, think about the fate of those 100 seeds you can water only once. Unless you have an unlimited source of water or marketing dollars you must think smaller to achieve greater results.

Don't let your ego get in the way... Target a smaller, focused area and you'll win every time.

Commit to marketing

A mediocre marketing program with a dedicated effort will always be more successful than an award-winning strategy that is executed halfheartedly. Dedication is the reason businesses and marketing efforts succeed. Show me a successful business of any kind, and I will show you a dedication to marketing. The flaw in most dental practices with regard to marketing is misunderstanding this important concept. Marketing is not an expense, marketing is an investment. If it is executed properly, every penny spent will return to you multiple times. To understand how I really feel about this philosophy, hopefully you've already read "The Parable of the Wise Fisherman" in the first chapter of this book.

If I had a dollar for every time I heard a dentist tell me

that he or she couldn't afford marketing, I'd be a rich man. When dentists start to see marketing like they see their dental supplies, they are headed in the right direction. When they start to see dental marketing like they see their retirement account, they are finally starting to get it.

Marketing is not an expense, it's an investment

Repeat, repeat, repeat

It takes a while for prospects to trust you, and if you change your marketing, media, and identity, you'll lose most of the investment spent to that point and essentially have to start over. Frequency and familiarity are important principles. Imagine if McDonald's only ran ads when sales were slow. Or, what if every time you saw a McDonald's ad it was entirely different, with no common theme or consistent message. If that was how it was done, two all-beef patties, special sauce, lettuce, cheese, pickles, onions on a sesame seed bun, wouldn't mean anything to you. The magic is, that it does.

Build your brand by telling the same story over and over.

Patience is a virtue

Marketing works. But, it takes a fair amount of time to really kick into high gear. You must be willing to stick it out and patiently wait for your seeds to grow. They say that the difference between hunters and farmers is just patience. Hunters eat what they kill. Hunters live for the moment. Hunters often go hungry and sometimes on rare occasions when hunting is good, they have an abundance and gorge themselves. Farmers on the other hand, must patiently wait for their crops to grow. They watch them very carefully and pray for their success. Hunters don't have the faith and long-term vision that farmers are required to have to be successful. When farming is executed properly, entire communities can be fed and as seed is re-invested each year, a multiple of that investment is returned at harvest time. Marketing is not at all different. You must live for tomorrow and plan accordingly.

Become a marketing farmer. Leave hunting to your competitors.

Variety is the spice of life

Your marketing strategy must include multiple tactics. In warfare, a one-dimensional effort rarely results in victory. Ground troops, air artillery, special forces, and every weapon imaginable are required to attack the enemy at every point. In dental marketing the same applies. Sometimes, all it takes is one postcard. Sometimes, it requires multiple tactics over a period of time to create the motivation for a new patient to call and schedule. As in warfare, your tactical weapons need to compliment each other to create an overall victory.

A one-dimensional marketing effort will result in a one-dimensional success.

Convenience

People now believe that time is not money, but is far more valuable than money. Respect this by being easy to do business with and running your company for the convenience of your customers not yourself. Ask yourself, "What would I want in a dentist." Also, notice what other businesses are doing to adopt the mentality that whatever the customer wants, the customer gets. And they get it, when and where it is convenient. Look at Kinkos. Consider Wal-Mart. Emulate Wendy's. These companies live for customer convenience.

Don't worry about your competition, emulate great convenience companies like Kinkos.

Word of mouth

It is a proven fact, that people are more likely to talk about your dental practice when they are unhappy, than when they are happy or satisfied. Good customer service can protect you from as much negative word-of-mouth as possible, but the real trick, is to get people talking positively about your practice.

People don't want to go to the telephone book to pick a lawyer. People don't want to pick a real-estate agent from the Yellow Pages–or an accountant, or a chiropractor, or an insurance agent, or most importantly a dentist. People want referrals! The only hurdle is linking the people who need your services with the patients who are likely to provide a referral. A structured word-of-mouth campaign begins by enabling your patients with tactical tools, that will make providing a referral easy to do. We'll discuss these tools later in another chapter.

Referrals cost very little, but failing to make them a priority can be very expensive.

Sell the sizzle

There are elements of your practice that you take for granted, but prospects would be amazed if they knew the details. Be sure all of your marketing always reflects that amazement. It's always there. For example, clear braces, digital x-rays with all of their advantages, same-day laser whitening, conscious sedation and on and on. Many dentists think the public doesn't care about what goes on behind the scenes and may find dental technology dull. Actually the opposite is true. The public loves new and exciting advances in medical treatment. Make sure you read more about my philosophy on "selling the sizzle" in the chapter on case presentation.

Everybody loves a bit of sizzle with their steak.

And sell the steak

Don't believe that old adage, "Sell the sizzle not the steak." Sophisticated patients these days know the style from the substance and won't buy into the style alone. You always have to back up your sizzle with a healthy serving of steak. The steak is great customer service, excellent dentistry, and a flawless patient experience. We'll get into more of that later.

Too much sizzle and not enough steak won't cut it anymore.

Can't buy me love

The Beatles had it right. Money can't buy you love and it can't buy patient loyalty. A relationship with a loyal patient over your entire career can be worth many thousands of dollars. Not only from that patient's own dental care and the dental care of their family, but from the referrals of friends and associates they may refer to you, if you've earned their business. No marketing campaign, no matter how well thought through and executed can make up for the loss of a great patient. It's like a leak in a bucket that keeps losing water no matter how fast you refill it. The leaks must be fixed before you can expect optimum results from your marketing efforts.

If you want patient loyalty, put away your wallet... you'll have to earn it the hard way.

Tracking your results

The final and most important marketing principle I want to drive home is tracking your results. Tracking is easy, but nobody can do it for you. The most effective marketing consultant in the world can't, and won't, be able to sit in your office, and do a formal head-count of new patients who respond to your marketing program. You can't miss phone calls, you can't expect patients to remind you how they heard about you, and you especially can't forget to tell your team you decided to run an ad.

To optimize marketing results, you must understand which marketing tactic is driving the best response, and whether new offers increase response versus previous efforts. You can only draw conclusive results, if you are willing to adopt tracking and measurement policies in your practice.

For example, most dentists make a note in the file of a new patient if they were referred by an existing patient and who it was. Unfortunately, most practices don't make a similar note in the file of the patient who gave the referral. It's an easy fix, and a powerful bit of information.

Any good marketing consultant will give you assistance in the best method to track your results. I think the best advice is to simply keep a list of where all new patients come from. It sounds sort of over simplified but it's not, and unfortunately few dentists make it a priority.

Ignorance is bliss, but track your marketing results anyway.

BRANDING DEMYSTIFIED

What is branding?

What is the single most important objective of the
marketing process? ... We believe it's the process of
branding. Marketing is building a brand in the mind of
the prospect. If you can build a powerful brand, you will
have a powerful marketing program. If you can't, then
all the advertising, fancy packaging, sales promotion
and public relations in the world won't help you achieve
your objective.'

– Al Ries And Laura Ries, 'World Class Brands'

It's easy to explain how Coke has become a brand after 100 years of advertising and marketing efforts, but sometimes, it is very difficult to explain how a dentist creates a brand with relatively few resources, in just one community, and in a short period of time.

It always starts with a great product, a great location, and a great in-office experience. However, many dental practices with all of these necessary requirements, (and they are all necessary) never really build a "brand." Something else must be required and I'm going to try to explain it in very simple terms in this chapter.

Many marketing experts talk about brands, but for this discussion, lets not be so concerned about brand building as we are building a loyal community of believers in your dental services. We may even refer to them as patriots, fans and advocates. As a dental professional, you may not relate to actually building a brand, but you *do* think a lot about the group of people that prefer your products and services—your patients.

In the simplest of terms, brand building can be boiled down to the fact that brands are belief systems. Once you think of a brand as a belief system, you automatically understand the things that giant companies spend billions of dollars trying to obtain: trust, quality, vision, values, leadership, and on and on.

Simply stated, brand building is just a fancy way to describe the job of creating loyalty.

Four simple steps

Building a brand for a dental practice can be broken into four simple steps. These steps are critical to brand building for any small service business, but they are a perfect plan for any dental professional to follow.

Number 1 is a creation story. Apple Computer is about a couple of guys who built personal computers in their parent's garage. Nike started with a guy making running shoes with a waffle iron. UPS was started by a fifteen year-old with a bicycle. Who are you?

Even if you don't have a personal creation story, where were you born? Where did you go to high school? Where did you go to dental school? Are you married? Kids? Do you love dogs?

Branding pioneer Jack Trout asserts that the creation story is critical, simply because that story "is often at the heart of being different and successful."

Number 2, what are you about? All belief systems have a creed that boldly claims what you believe in. Do you think different? Do you have any special training that influences your treatment philosophy? Do you provide an extra level of service, or do you provide any products and services that other dentists don't?

Number 3. Once we know where you're from and what you're about, show us who you are. All great brands have visual icons or symbols that sum up who they are and what they're about. The Nike swoosh. The Stars and Stripes. The Olympic Rings. Icons are not just logos and images, but they spark the other senses as well. The taste of McDonald's French fries, the smell of BMW leather trim, the feel of a Tommy Bahama silk shirt, and the Coca Cola jingles we've all memorized.

Number 4. Every powerful brand has a set of sacred words that are associated with the product or service. These sacred words are found in every component of the brand's packaging, advertising, and sales literature. The sacred words are constantly on the lips of every member of the corporate team. They are spoken by celebrity voices and show up at sports arenas, airports and the pages of Time Magazine. We believe the sacred words because they become a part of our subconscious and part of the fabric of our society.

Build a brand in four easy steps. It sounds like an infomercial but it works.

The branding steps at work

Take Coke. The creation story is about Dr. John Pemberton creating a carbonated drugstore beverage. The creed is about "the real thing." The icons are the shapely bottle profile and the Coke red ribbon. The sacred words include "Coke", "It's the real thing", "Coke is it", and other words exclusive to the Coke experience.

Or the iPod. The creation story has to do with bringing Steve Jobs back into the Apple empire and the redesign of personal computing and Apple Corp. The creed is about delivering sound and pictures in portable ways like no other company has ever tried. The icons are the elegant design of the iPod and the striking two-color ads. The sacred words are the product names that surrounds the "i" universe - iPod, iTunes, iPhoto—a hip, naming convention that followers have stolen.

Is it working? Do Diet Coke drinkers get upset on the airline when they find that they only serve Pepsi products? Try taking an iPod away from its owner and replacing it with a Sony MP3 player.

When people believe, they belong. When they belong to the group that surrounds your dental services, they are willing to refer friends and family to your practice. Remember the last time you moved? Where did you find out about the best grocery store? The best church? The auto mechanic who wouldn't rip you off? Probably from someone who already "belonged" to their group, someone who preferred them above all others and was willing to advocate that preference.

Branding is a process that can help you position your dental products and services by creating a community of people to surround them. Brands are built by providing products and services that people can believe in.

If you want to understand branding, study Coke and Apple Computer.

Don't become another generic dentist

To the general public it can be difficult to differentiate one dentist from another. This difficulty has been magnified for decades, by dentists who offer no special competitive advantage or unique approach to dentistry. The shame is that with the cutting edge equipment, procedures, and high tech dental philosophies in place, it isn't very hard to be special. Especially, since only a small percentage of the dentists in the industry seem to understand the unique opportunity that is before them.

Update your old equipment. Become comfortable with cosmetic dentistry. Invest in a laser and digital radiography. Spend some money perfecting your front office with one of the many invaluable patient education systems available. Hire a practice management coach and perfect your craft. Then, when you have done these things and more, shout it from the top of your roof!

Consumers are always looking for something special... Make your practice special.

Be number two

One of the most powerful places your dental practice can be is number #2 in your market. What I mean, is that many potential patients in your community already have some type of a relationship with a dentist. The relationships in many cases may even go back many years and seem healthy and strong. However, as soon as a patient has a bad enough experience, or perhaps a their dentist retires, they start looking for a replacement to their existing dentist. It may be a raise in fees, a rude office manager, or any number of negative issues. When this happens, you want to be positioned as the number one alternative to their existing dentist. This is a tactic that is used very effectively by many of the best salesmen in the world. Brand yourself well, keep your nose clean, provide the best care, and wait for the competition to make a mistake. Then move-in.

Be number two in your market and you'll never need new patients.

Marketing to women and their daughters

According to recent studies by major market research firms, 63% of online shoppers are women. Women control 75% of household finances and 80% of purchasing decisions. Women buy or influence the purchase of 80% of all consumer goods. Women also influence 85% of all health care decisions.

Do you see the opportunity here? If not, you might as well stop reading this section right now. But if you realize how lucrative addressing the needs of women in the dental world can be, then you'll need to understand what influences their purchasing decisions.

As we all know, men and women are different. We respond differently to the same communication and social situations. A man and woman listening to the same conversation might come away with completely different impressions of what was said.

For example: men tend to choose a dentist based mostly on price and convenience, women utilize a more careful approach. Your receptionist's tone of voice, or the photo in your yellow page ad might not matter to a man, but might be a deciding factor for a woman. Why? Women are more likely to make buying decisions based not only on the dental services you provide, but on what your practice stands for. This once again reinforces women's relationship approach to purchasing. So, if you want to attract women, become focused on softer features and benefits that are important to them—and make sure your marketing message communicates it loud and clear.

The premise behind this reality is simple: If women have to go out of their way to track you down... if you make them jump through hoops to get service... if your attitude is take-it-or leave it... they'll probably leave it—and take their dental dollars elsewhere. Your objective with female customers should be built on a long-term reputation of honesty, integrity, ethical behavior, and "off-the-charts" attention to detail. And most importantly, always remember that it's easier to keep her than to win her back.

Women are not afraid to stop and ask for help, so they will respond more to quality customer service standards and a polished office flow than any of their male counterparts. And even though men may not be as in need of these intangibles, if you incorporate the higher standards of women into your practice, you are bound to give men a bit more than they even thought to ask for.

And finally, studies have also shown that graphic design and advertising that uses cliché women's colors (pinks and purples) or focus on "women's topics," will always alienate male patients. Women can also feel turned-off by such an obvious approach as well.

Women get it. Men don't... but who cares?

IMAGE IS EVERYTHING

Image is everything

When building a dental practice—and struggling with patients, cash-flow and employees, focusing on artsy matters might seem like a huge distraction. But as any celebrity publicist will tell you, *image is everything, baby!* That doesn't mean you need to be developing detailed brand marketing campaigns when what you really need in the short run are a few more patients. But it does mean you need to pay attention to things like your company name, logo and basic marketing materials, such as your Internet site. It also means that you'll have to focus on the image of your facility, your equipment and even your own teeth.

To begin the process of creating the perfect image for your practice, think about your patients' priorities. Do they most value speed, quality or price? If the potential patients in your demographic area appreciate quality above the other two attributes, your marketing plan and image should reflect this—right down to selecting a name. If, on the other hand, you believe your ideal patient values cheerful service above speed and price, everything about your image should embody those priorities. Their core values should be reflected in your customer-service policy, your logo, Internet site, signage, and every "touch-point" your patient has with your practice.

Make sure your shoes are shined and your socks match. Image is everything!

JetBlue

For an example of a real image success story, let's examine JetBlue. When the airline began operations, the price of its fares put it squarely in the low-budget category when it first took flight in 2000. Yet in just a few short years, and with a few clever image-building techniques, JetBlue has managed to elevate its company's image from "cheap" to "cheap chic." By using catchy language to describe everything from its travel map to its customer comment box, JetBlue manages to say to the public that, like its young, Web-savvy customers, it is smart, edgy and irreverent. With everything JetBlue does—its design elements, its press releases—you're getting the impression that JetBlue is fun, hip, fresh, and cool. What a great image.

JetBlue gets it. Do you?

What's in a name?

Because so many dental practices want positive and cosmetic words in their names—like esthetic, prestige, superior and elite—you might have a hard time coming up with something unique. Businesses all over the country feel that same pressure. That's why so many of them now resort to creating completely new words for company names, like Equitex, Immucell and Genitope. Others modify, misspell or combine words to create their names—like Cingular, Tekknowledge and Featherlite. Or they pick a common word that's unrelated to their business but carries positive associations, like Apple Computer. A dental practice with an original name such as Sundance Dental Center, or Pinnacle Oral Care will be so much easier to build a brand around, and position as a premier dental care facility than Smith Family Dental.

Beware of geographical names. Unless you want your business to be tied to a specific location—like Gainesville Family Dental or Abilene Oral Institute, you should choose a name that gives your company room to grow into new towns or cities. At some point you might want to explore new markets. Don't pick a name that holds you back.

Pick your friends and the name of your practice very carefully.

But, I like my name

Another naming issue facing many dental practices is the decision to use the name of the dentist. When a practice has been known as Anderson Dental Care for twenty years it becomes very tricky for Dr. Robert

Anderson to sell his practice to Dr. Mariah Woo. This is an example of good branding of a practice backfiring. For dentists that are currently in this situation, begin now to downplay your name. This can be accomplished by combining a new practice name with your own name for a while and then slowly subordinating your name over time. It can be tricky but it is very necessary to build long-term brand value. By the way, this process may take several years to make it as subtle as possible so begin now.

I like my name too. But, not for my company.

Cheesy logos

I cannot stress this concept strongly enough. LOSE THE CORNY AND CHEESY LOGOS! The public in the 21st century is a very sophisticated buying audience. The image of the Mr. Tooth logo, and the tooth flexing his cavity-fighting muscles, is tired and old. Avoid anything cartoony, silly or funny. Those kinds of messages will never help you create a brand as a superior dental professional. I won't dwell any longer on this section.

Enough said.

Your walls

I love fly fishing. I also love artwork of southern Utah where I'm from. However, making these images part of my wall decor says nothing about the marketing services I provide. Likewise, the walls of your dental practice are not extensions of your personal life. Make your walls count for something and very purposely use dental imagery and dental messages to support the image you are building.

Another mistake I see all too often, is a dental practice with either bare walls or a complete disregard for image because the walls are cluttered with tacky dental posters and framed statements of their financial policies. Be careful. You probably have a fair amount of patients who make a living as interior designers, marketing executives, architects or real estate developers. Believe me, these individuals are sensitive to image and notice everything–good or bad.

Treat your walls like premium advertising space–because They are.

Your reception area

Just as your walls are important to your image, your reception area is also–maybe even more important. It never ceases to amaze me when I do a magazine count in some practices. I've seen as many as fifty magazines at a time piled on an end table or even worse hanging on the wall. This tells me that patients are spending entirely too long waiting for their appointment. It also tells me that somebody is afraid to throw away a six month old copy of People Magazine. Keep magazines to a minimum. Maybe six or seven. And make sure they are in good condition and current.

If possible a patient or parent of a patient should have a chance to read about advancements in cosmetic dentistry or read a patient brochure about your new laser or implant system. Another powerful tool is DVD–and, I don't mean Shrek or Star Wars. Several companies including my own, have created beautiful DVD presentations that are designed to be played on a continuous loop in the reception area. In the case of our DVD, it can be played with no sound, and includes beautiful scenery, imagery of smiling people and families, as well as 3-D animated dental education content. It is incredibly impressive when played on a large plasma screen display. Systems like this will communicate to your patients in dramatic fashion, that image and technology is a top priority.

You never get a second chance to make a first impression.

Leveraging giants

Pay careful attention to this short section. It will have a very positive effect on your image and brand. Dozens of dental companies spend hundreds of millions every year promoting their products to dentists. These companies have all produced sales and educational literature for patients. They are usually free to use or cost very little. In fact, some of them have started advertising direct to the public in an attempt to further drive their brand recognition. As I will mention later in this book, dentists who marry these brands with their own, will differentiate themselves and seem much more than just another generic dental practice. For example, when discussing an implant case with a patient, make your implant system of choice part of the discussion. "Mary, in our practice we use a new implant system from a company called ***Acme Dental Implants***. They have created a wonderful new technology that will make your new teeth look amazing." or "Steve, we have recently been introducing a new technology to our patients that lets us place metal free crowns that look just like natural teeth. It's a system developed by ***John Doe Technologies***, and it's called ***Great Product***." I have left out specific brand names but I think you see how easy it can be.

Whether in the actual case presentation or as part of

your marketing literature, Internet site or your walls, leveraging these huge brands as part of your own brand image will have a significant effect on your success.

Take a ride on their coat tails. It's free!

A great location

W e've all heard the old real estate axiom. Location, Location, Location. In dentistry as in most businesses this rule applies. Here's why. Great signage and foot traffic can be a huge part of not only image-building, but basic new-patient flow. I've seen practices with great locations do very little or no external marketing and still have a healthy number of new patients every week. I've also seen the opposite happen. A dumpy little practice on a backstreet with poor visibility and the new patient flow is almost non-existent. If I were building a new practice today I would find an area of town with the most foot traffic, parking and visibility. Many of the new strip malls around the country fit this bill and showcase modern construction and upper-end retailers. The lease space is always more costly, but the image, exposure and foot traffic are priceless. On the other hand the opposite advice applies. Stay away from the rundown retail strips with liquor stores and check-cashing outlets. You know what I mean.

Location. Location. Location. It never gets old.

Your own teeth!

It never ceases to amaze me when I see a dentist with crappy teeth. What gives? It can't be anything other than ignorance. Please look in the mirror and if you need to whiten or straighten or veneer or whatever, take care of it! When it comes to not practicing what you preach, a dentist with bad breath is also another dead giveaway. If you don't care, why should your patients?

Look in the mirror once in awhile.

CUSTOMER SERVICE IS NOT A DEPARTMENT

Become obsessed with customer service

If a dental practice did nothing else but become obsessed with customer service a lot of other problems would solve themselves. As the saying goes, "Customer service is dead." Our society has become completely devoid of great experiences between businesses and customers. Convenience and speed have trumped everything else.

This lack of expectation, however, gives dentists an opportunity to exceed expectations and stand out as a bright light in a dark world of customer frustration.

While in your office, or on the phone, make each patient feel like they are the single most important person in your practice. Accommodate their busy lives by being available anytime, anywhere. Memorize their names. Get to know their families. Know what they do for a living. Reward them handsomely for referring friends and families. Spoil their children with attention. Offer them a refreshment. Give them a hot towel before they leave. Hug them. Hold their hand. Rub their backs. Do whatever you have to make their customer experience awesome. You can't buy the loyalty that will come from your efforts.

Your patients are like the goose that lays golden eggs. Make sure they feel like it.

Their last impression may be their only impression

An otherwise great customer experience followed up with even a small negative experience with insurance or finances, will strain any relationship you've tried hard to build. One bad recall experience may undermine a long-term friendship with an old patient. A 30 minute wait in the chair for a dentist who is on the phone with a supplier, may alter the future of what could have been a loyal patient and his or her multiple referrals.

Make their last impression the best impression

Who answers the phone?

I want to make this point as clearly as I can. Don't let anyone answer your phone that hasn't got a great phone voice and a friendly disposition! I have called hundreds of offices over the years and it never ceases to amaze me how many monotone or even grumpy individuals, become that practices first impression. It speaks volumes for the rest of the practice, whether accurate or not.

On the other hand, I have watched the right person on the phone with the right personality, diffuse even the most difficult situations and win the friendship of the most bitter patients.

If you've got a receptionist or any other team member who can be grumpy from time to time, or has the attitude that it is her job to protect the practice from less-than-perfect patients, make a change today! Don't put it off another moment.

You spent a small fortune getting your dental degree and probably even more setting up your practice. You've got a lot invested and you have a huge responsibility to be successful. The person answering the phone and greeting patients is your gate-keeper to the world. Don't mess it up.

You can't afford not to have the right person answering the phone

The science of the phone

The telephone is your link to the outside world. Not only is the person who answers the phone very important, but the number of phones you have, the hours of the day you answer the phone, your answering service or machine and even how many phone lines you have are all critical to phone success. I have a good friend named Steve Sperry that is nationally recognized as a dental expert and coach. Among many other things, Steve helps dental practices see the phone in their office as a powerful marketing tool. He also shows dentists how often they have obvious holes in their telephone tactics. Steve teaches, that the telephone must be answered five days a week by a real person at the practice. This doesn't mean that the practice has to see patients everyday, but having a recorded message on Friday or during lunch hours is risky. It's risky, because phone studies have shown that peak calling hours are on Friday and also during the lunch hour. The main reason for these peak times is that people who work are available more often during those times. Another peak begins Monday morning at 7:00 am.

Perfecting the way you handle inbound phone calls is critical to the success of an overall marketing plan. If you don't understand the phones or you don't have the right processes in place, an otherwise great marketing plan, can suffer from an "easy-to-fix," weak link in the chain.

How much does it really cost a practice that fails on the phone? The world may never know.

The right team

I probably hear on a weekly basis, from a dentist I am working with, that he or she is unhappy with one or more members of their dental team. I always laugh and ask them why they don't make a change. The answers are always based on fear. Fear of change, fear of failure to handle the extra work load, fear of an emotional mess, fear of this and fear of that. It has been my experience, over many years, working with many employees, that people rarely change and that creating the right team may require some uncomfortable changes before finding great people.

However, before you run out and fire your whole team like some of you would like to do, make sure that *you* aren't the problem. Great leadership is required to create a great practice. I won't go into any leadership advice at this point because others are more qualified to give it. My only advice would be to look in the mirror every so often, and ask yourself how *you* can be easier to work with.

Once you have assembled a great team hang on to them! Don't get cocky and don't get greedy. A great team that is firing on all eight cylinders will be the most important asset you create as a dentist. Great teams are the exception to the rule. I don't say that to make you afraid that you'll never have the right team. Every dentist can do it if they make it a priority and play by the rules of the game. And, the number one rule is to make an emotional investment in the success of every team member. This investment comes in the form of top pay for top production, important benefits such as health care, mutual respect, and frequent and sincere thank-you's, expressed openly in the presence of other team members. Entire books have been written on this topic and I would recommend that every dentist becomes a student of the science of creating great teams and working environments.

A great team is the single most important asset in your practice.

Training

Great teams need great training. Take advantage of the many resources that are available to dental practices for team training. Whether the training is clinical or otherwise, your team members will begin to understand the value you place on them being their best. Yes, it can be expensive and yes, it takes away from production time. However, it will pay huge dividends in the long run that will far outweigh the short term investment.

The only caveat I would give you, is to confirm for yourself that your team is ready to commit themselves for more than a few months, before you make any investment in training. The last thing you want to do is foot the bill for their next employer's training.

Pay for training now, or pay for it in other less pleasant ways later. The choice is yours.

Thank you! Thank you!

Patients who refer to your practice should be thanked, and I mean more than just a handshake and a slap on the back. Blow the dust off your wallet and spend a few bucks on such a great patient. Whether it is movie tickets, fresh flowers, a dinner on you, or something like a box of Omaha Steaks sent to their home on dry ice. Fifty dollars spent here and there on the right patients is a powerful practice building tactic. My company has developed an easy and convenient way to send a great gift package to your patients that you can access at our website at www.idmtools.com. The way you do it doesn't matter. Just make sure you do it.

When possible, send the gift to your patient's place of work. Imagine the impact a half-dozen fresh roses would have on not only your patient, but their co-workers. It makes you remarkable.

Now there's an image builder!

Pick up the pace

Convenience and speed are everything today. It used to be that the idea of an overnight package was almost hard to believe. Now the only time we overnight something, is when we're not in a hurry. Instead of letters we have e-mail. A roll of film used to take a week to develop. Next, it was same-day, then one-hour developing. Now, we have digital cameras. And , it's not stopping. Learn to work fast in all areas of your practice. I don't mean to rush procedures or lower your standard of quality. And, I especially don't mean to eliminate the personal touch because you're in a hurry. What I mean is, make patient forms easier to deal with by making them available at your website so they can be filled out before the patient even arrives. Perfect the flow and scheduling to eliminate waiting. Invest in dental technology that will speed up x-rays or imaging or whatever. Get your lab to shorten their delivery schedule. Most labs can turn around a crown in three or four days. They just have a bad habit of taking as much time as you'll give them. The list can get quite lengthy. Suffice it to say that time is the most important commodity in our crazy society. Make sure you're on the winning end of it.

It's a tired old saying but it's still profound. Time is money.

Crawl through broken glass

The title of this heading says it all. If you and your team will maintain such enthusiasm for customer service that you'd be willing to crawl through broken glass to keep a patient, you're right where you need to be.

It will only bleed for a while.

PUBLIC RELATIONS

Keep in touch

One of the reasons dentists lose patients is because they do a poor job of staying in touch with their customers. The corporate world calls this a "touch-point." Companies like America Online and General Motors spend millions on creating better ways to maintain frequent communication with their customers. In fact, in many ways it is becoming very elaborate and very personalized.

In a dental practice, recall usually makes up the entire process of creating a "touch-point." Instead of just recall, I recommend that dentists mail a personalized letter on a quarterly basis. Newsletters have also been effective although they require a major time investment. I have found that a short personalized letter is more effective and more affordable. A personal follow-up with patients who have recently been treated is extremely effective and can have more of an impact when the dentist makes the call himself or herself. Recall made by the dentist when appropriate or possible can have a profound success on re-activating patients that aren't responding to other team members. There are many creative and unique ways of creating "touch-points;" just make sure you start doing something now. You can get innovative later.

Giant corporations spend millions "keeping in touch." Make sure you follow their lead.

Recall cards

Recall cards can be effective if they are used correctly, but I have a concern with some aspects of the concept. Here's why: They can become an excuse for not making phone calls, and certain card designs can border on being too cheesy. For example, the jack-o'-lantern with braces on its teeth and the worm in the apple holding a toothbrush have got to go! Your recall cards need to be sophisticated and educational and they need to match your overall brand image. Don't let them replace your personal phone calls, and make sure they are sent out consistently.

Recall cards are effective if they look great and are implemented properly.

Testimonials

Although patient testimonials should be included in every part of your marketing plan, I have included them in this chapter because they are such an important part of your public opinion and image. Testimonials for your practice are easy to get and should always be updated and added to. I don't have to tell you when you should ask for a written testimonial from a patient. You'll know it when it happens. The perfect patient and the perfect case. Make sure you take pictures of your work, as you should for many of your cases and ask the patient to record in a sentence or two how they felt about their experience at your practice. These testimonials can be used as wall art, on direct mail cards, at your website and practice brochure. They are invaluable as a marketing component and will make your marketing experts job much easier. If you don't feel comfortable asking a patient for a brief testimonial, get over it. You can't afford to let your own feelings to get in the way of such a necessary public relations message.

Keep testimonials brief and make sure to take pictures of the patient and your work.

Press releases

From time to time I'll have a dentist ask me about press releases. For those of you who don't know what a press release is and how they work, let me explain it as simply as I can.

A press release or news release is a written or recorded communication directed at members of the news media for the purpose of announcing something claimed as having news value. Typically, it is mailed or faxed to assignment editors at newspapers, magazines, radio stations, television stations, and/or television networks. Commercial news wire services are also used to distribute news releases. Press releases are sent for the purpose of announcing press conferences, breaking news, financial announcements, sports scores and on and on.

Even for large companies, press releases are sometimes hard to control. News agencies are so bombarded by "news" that getting noticed is extremely difficult. To facilitate this process, public relations firms can be retained to do the hard work and push your information through the system. Every dollar I've ever spent on a PR firm I wished I could get back. It is a business that I really don't believe in because I've never seen the return on investment that is hoped for.

The attraction for most small businesses and dental practices, to be specific, is free exposure. Unfortunately, it's usually never free. Most news and media companies give most exposure to paying advertisers. Many magazines and newspapers will package a feature story or article with an advertising contract to sweeten the deal. Like they say, nothing is free.

I know a dentist in Salt Lake City that was able to arrange for a short segment on a morning television news show. The show featured his new soft tissue laser and specifically his ability to treat canker sores and cold sores with some success. The news crew showed up and it was quite a good production. He spent a lot of time arranging for the opportunity and after all was said and done, he picked up three or four patients, but the return was hardly worth the investment of time.

My advice to dentists, is to focus on targeted marketing efforts that can be measured and controlled. A press release is a tricky proposition. If you can get it without a lot of work, by all means go for it. However, I would never recommend that a concentrated effort be made. Most of the time it's great for the ego but not for the bank account.

Press release are great if they fall in your lap. But don't spend much time trying to get one.

ADVERTISING TACTICS THAT WORK

and a few that don't.

Direct mail

The single most effective marketing tactic to create new patient flow is direct mail. Believe me, I've tried them all and nothing "pulls" quite like a direct mail campaign that is well executed. The problem that dentists have from time to time with direct mail is that they do it wrong. Direct mail is not as simple as flinging a postcard into a few thousand mailboxes and watching the new patients lining up at your door.

Another misconception with direct mail marketing is that 1% is an acceptable return. Somewhere, in some twenty year old marketing text book, this statistic stuck in everybody's mind. The truth is, 1% is a home run. In fact, 1% is out-of-the-park. A more realistic number for dental direct mail marketing is .020% to .035%. That means that a 10,000 piece direct mail campaign should result in 20-35 new patients. However, a 1% return would be 100 patients. Although a 1% return is not unheard of, it's a safer bet to expect something less.

Now, I have seen results approaching 1%, however, those results are never the norm. It's kind of like the diet commercials that promise 50 lbs. of weight loss in sixty days. It's possible, but not likely. Typically, such results are seen in markets that are growing rapidly and everyone is looking for a dentist. Las Vegas comes to mind.

Direct mail has to be executed precisely to be effec.
The quality of the printing and design, the mailing
list, the offer, and the timing are just a few important
considerations. Do it right, and it will become the
foundation for the rest of your marketing tactics.

***Next to $100 bills with every cleaning, direct
mail is the most effective way to beat the
competition.***

E-mail

Although e-mail is a cool way to externally market a
dental practice it is difficult for dentists. Here's why;
most practices don't have their patients' email addresses!
We live in the computer and information age. Everyone
uses instant messaging, the internet and e-mail. Please do
yourself a huge favor and begin collecting your patients
email addresses today. For just a few dollars a month you
can send a sophisticated e-newsletter. For almost nothing
you can send every patient a hip and fun electronic
birthday card or an electronic coupon for free whitening.
With email you can easily keep your patients updated on
your latest technology improvements and advancements
in dentistry. Companies like mine make it very easy and
can help you manage the whole process in just minutes.

***E-mail is the most affordable and effective way
to maintain frequent contact with every patient.***

Internet sites

I hate to even put Internet sites in the advertising chapter, because they are more effective as an image builder and patient communication tool. The simple fact is, the general public isn't searching the Internet for a good dentist. That's not just my opinion. It's a documented statistic that any one with access to the Internet can get. Internet marketers have tried for years to make websites a viable advertising tactic for business that operate in a regionalized area. So far, their results have been poor at best. Dry cleaners, auto repair, restaurants, chiropractors, and yes even dental practices are service businesses with a very local target market when compared to companies that have national markets. In fact, most dentists should only target the consumers within five miles of their facility which further complicates a dental Internet strategy.

In my opinion, Internet marketing companies that promise high numbers of new patients to dentists who purchase a site from them are scam artists. The Internet is complicated and foreign to most dentists and they are an easy target. The only way to predict your exposure using the Internet is through pay-per-click advertising. "PPC" ads only cost the advertiser if an Internet user clicks on the ad for more information. However, PPC ads have a fatal flaw. Anybody can click on your ad, including another dentist or your office manager, and you still pay for the click. And as I've stated already, Internet advertising will never make sense for a dentist until a larger number of individuals are actually using the internet to find a new dentist.

Now, don't get me wrong. An Internet site is vitally important part of a comprehensive marketing plan. It's a great way to improve your image, educate your patients and provide information for individuals who have received one of your printed marketing pieces. My company builds great websites, and we believe they are a necessary part of doing business in our society. However, don't be fooled. As a stand-alone advertising medium, websites are weak.

The public in general is not using the Internet to find a new dentist.

Television

When I see dentists advertising on television I wonder how they were ever fooled into such a crazy stunt. Television is great for consumer products, major brands, informercials and goods and services that are sold on a large scale. For local service providers like dentists, television has way too much reach. The demographics are difficult to target and it can be very expensive.

To make it even worse, people are so jaded to television commercials that you're fighting a losing battle from the start. The remote control is your worst enemy. We've been trained to flip the channel using the remote control as soon as a commercial comes on. Unlike a printed ad piece, television vaporizes in 30 seconds. If the prospect doesn't take the time to write down your phone number you've lost your opportunity to connect with the consumer.

Next time you see a 30 second ad on TV for a dentist, whose practice is 20 miles away, ask yourself if you would run to the phone and call. I think I already know your answer.

Radio

Radio is a lot like television. Way too much reach is the main problem. The only saving grace for radio is the ability to increase the frequency over television simply due to the higher cost of TV compared to radio. However, that being said, in some major markets radio can be as much as $500 for one spot during morning drive time. Radio ads are also much easier to create than TV ads. Still, I'd stick with what has proven to be effective, and radio usually isn't it.

For dentists, the only advertising worse than radio is TV.

Billboards and outdoor ads

The other day I got a good laugh when I saw an ad for a dentist on a park bench. The ad looked great, except for the part that was covered up by a drunk that had passed out on the bench. I could almost make out the phone number but the last two digits were covered up by his boots. I like outdoor ads that are close to the practice and are seen mostly by local residents. Ads on smaller streets or on roads that enter or exit a town or community can be very effective.

On the other hand, giant billboards on main Interstate freeways may be great for the ego of the dentist but usually create a less than desirable response. As in all good advertising tactics, outdoor advertising needs to make an impact and must be offer-based to get attention. Make sure you work with a professional to get the best results. Never do it yourself.

Outdoor advertising can be tricky. Start out small and test your results carefully.

Yellow pages

I hate yellow pages advertising. There, I've said it. It's out of my system and I feel OK to continue. My hate for this type of advertising stems from the horror stories

I've come across over the years where dentists have lost thousands of dollars, and years out of their practices, after being waltzed down the path of failure by Yellow Pages companies.

Depending on its size and location, a Yellow Pages ad can cost up to $40,000 per year. With that same budget, a dentist could go crazy with a direct mail campaign and have many times the return. Unfortunately, by the time dentists realize their mistake they have committed to a long-term contract and have no budget left.

Depending on the size of your market, you may be competing with dozens or even hundreds of dentists who are all making the same claims and even using the same photography and graphic design. It is always interesting to see the ads the graphic designers at the Yellow Page companies come up with. They obviously have no real understanding of dental marketing and the dentist usually ends up controlling the look and message of the ad. Need I say more?

Once you place an ad, you have to wait a year to make any change to your ad. Mistakes or poor reproduction of photography are locked in. If you missed the target in any way, you've wasted a year. If you insist on utilizing Yellow Page ads, at least hire a dental marketing professional to help you put your best foot forward.

I'll say it again. I hate Yellow Pages advertising.

Coupon mailers

The biggest problem with coupons is image, or lack thereof. Who wants to advertise their practice along with baby diapers and carpet cleaning? Yes, I know even dentists clip coupons, we all do to some extent, but it's about the psychology of it all. I've worked with several dentists who swore by coupon stuffers. You see, the thing is, their image reflected it. And, nothing I could say would change their opinion.

You'll never see an ad for a Mercedes or a Rolex in a coupon mailer and there's a simple reason for it. Those companies flock with the eagles, not the pigeons. Do the same in your practice.

Magazines

Magazine ads can be great. They can also be a waste of money. My experience has shown me, that in addition to the ad needing to follow the basic rules for good ad design, the magazine itself is the real issue. (no pun intended) Magazines with a paid subscription and of course, a local audience can get a great response. Magazine are usually very demographic specific. Magazines usually have a good "shelf-life", that is, they stay on a coffee table for quite awhile. I know this because I see five year old copies of Time magazine in most dental offices. And, in most cases the right magazine can help you to be associated with other exclusive advertisers. Picking a magazine is a very regional matter and may be difficult for a marketing consultant to help choose. However, when I am asked to help a dental client create a magazine ad, I always like to see a copy of the magazine beforehand. Sometimes it's just gut feel. Other times, recommendations are made on circulation and other statistics provided by the publisher. Be very careful of committing to lengthy contracts. Ad salespeople love contracts and use discounts as the carrot. With some negotiation, you can usually get the same discount without the long-term commitment.

On a recent flight to New York I saw an ad in the United Airlines in-flight magazine for a dentist in Georgia. Not only did the ad break every marketing rule in book, but it reached an international audience of travelers. To the credit of the practice, they've helped raise the awareness of cosmetic dentistry for every passenger who sees the ad. The problem for the practice that paid the giant bill, is that local dentists in communities all over the world are the real benefactors. Those lucky dentists should send the practice in Georgia a thank-you note and a copy of this book.

Magazine ads can be a good investment, but chose the publication carefully.

Newspapers

Newspapers are a lot like magazines, in that results can be extremely dependent on the quality of the publication. I think that newspapers in small communities are a better bet than large newspapers. I also like Sunday issues. They have a better readership and people tend to spend time digesting them slowly. In general, I think newspapers are becoming less viable over time. As consumers we are all so bombarded by marketing messages, that an ad has to jump out and grab you by the hair. Newspapers are almost always black and white and the print quality is poor. My advice would be to test an ad or two. See what happens. Direct mail is such a powerful weapon that most other forms of print ads leave me a little cold.

On a scale of 1 to 10, I give newspapers a solid 4.

Other wacky stuff

I created this section to deal with everything else. For example, don't advertise in the playbill at the local junior high production of The Wizard of Oz. Don't advertise on the shopping carts at the liquor store. Don't advertise on park benches. (I covered that already) Don't advertise on pharmacy bags. Don't advertise in a Portuguese newspaper for Portuguese immigrants if you don't speak Portuguese (That's a true story). Don't send your team around town with door hangers and windshield flyers. In short, be a professional.

If you think it may look tacky, it probably will.

PATIENT ATTRITION

What is patient attrition

As I've already mentioned in this book, my partner is a practicing dentist. When he read this chapter he was concerned that as I discussed the term of attrition, dental professionals would think I was talking about worn down teeth. I had to laugh at his comment and it made me think that, actually, in many ways my idea of patient attrition is very much like teeth that become worn over time. First, let me clarify the terminology. When I say patient attrition, I am describing a shrinking patient base, and not shrinking teeth.

Sometimes the attrition of patient numbers is slow and subtle, and it doesn't seem to be causing any real issues today or even tomorrow; but, if the problem goes unchecked or untreated, it can cause much more serious issues as time passes. Just like a patient with an ever worsening dental condition, dental practices can find themselves in a real predicament as their patient numbers slowly dwindle without having a plan for replenishing the loss.

In this chapter I'll try to help you understand, simply and plainly, that patient attrition happens to every practice whether you like it or not, and that having a plan in place to replace lost patients is abosultely critical to the long-term viability of your practice.

It's worse than you think

Experienced dental consultants almost always agree that the patient attrition rate of an established practice runs between 10 and 12 percent each year, and that the attrition rate for patients in a new practice is in the 15 to 20 percent range. It occurs with every dentist and you can't stop it. Life happens. People move and people die. You can have every mechanism in place to prevent some type of patient loss, but in many ways it's not something you can control. Obviously, just to maintain status quo, you must attract at least as many new patients into your practice as you lose. Although the concept is simple, too many dentists don't accurately assess the number of lost patients when they determine their needs for new-patient flow. If you don't believe me, here are several reasons that patients leave a practice that are indisputable and based on national data and statistics.

Patients move

For years I've heard different statistics about the percentage of people that move each year. In every community it is different and the estimates vary from a low of 10 percent to a high of 25 percent. Using the information provided to the public by the U.S. Census Bureau, I'll try to simplify and clarify any confusion. Out of a population of 282,556,000 people in 2003, 40,093,000 moved. That's an overall percentage of 14.19 percent annually. These 40-plus-million people break down as follows:

- **23,468,000 moved within the same county**

- **7,728,000 moved to a different county in-state**

- **7,628,000 moved to a different state**

- **1,269,000 moved to a different country**

The major moving activity takes place within the 18-34 year olds, with people in their 20s representing the highest concentration. Once people reach their 50s, the move rate is minimal. And, in people over the age of 70, the move percentages are below 2 percent annually.

Couples with young children are the most likely to move a long distance. As people get older, the percentage who move decreases consistently. There are two exceptions to this trend. When people reach age 65, there is an increase in both the percentage of moves, and distance of the move. These statistics are likely due to retirement. When people reach age 85-plus, there is an increase in the percentage of moves, and a decrease in the distance of the move. This is possibly due to a move to an assisted living facility or long-term care center. As you read these statistics, I'm sure that you are already mentally comparing these numbers to your own patient base. From the many dentists I've discussed these numbers with, the data seems to be a fairly accurate reflection of what happens in a typical dental practice.

A patient moving out of an area is a reality for every dental practice, and it is important to remember that (more than likely) just one household can eliminate several patients. It is also important to remember that you'll never know about all of them. In fact, statistics confirm that half of the population moves without ever notifying the US Postal Service.

Patients die

As with population statistics of people who move, statistics of people who die each year is reported differently from various sources. However, for these statistics, I'll rely on the National Center for Health, which seem to be the most reputable and accurate. In 2003 the population of the United States was approximately 282,556,000. Out of such a population, 2,517,000 people will die each year. That's nearly one percent annually. It might not sound like a lot but in some practices that can be as many as 20 patients each year. It's a terrible topic to write about, but no practice is immune to the reality of individuals passing on.

Patients divorce

In 2003, there were a total of 1,214,990 divorces granted in the US. According to national divorce statistics, the average family unit affected by divorce included 3.14 members. Therefore, the total number of immediate family members affected by divorce was 3,816,068, or 1.3 percent of the population that year. Even if all family members remain in their community, the emotional distraction and change in financial means can keep those affected away from the dentist for long periods of time.

Patients file for bankruptcy

Each year in the United States one half of one percent (.5%) of the population files for some form of bankruptcy protection. Undoubtedly, these patients may be forced to place little or no emphasis on dental care, at least temporarily. As of the publishing date of this book, mortgage forclosure rates are at an all-time high. This is due in large part to the high number of adjustable rate mortgages and other flexible loan structures. In fact, in 2006 forclosure were up 45% over the previous year.

Patients get Cancer

Each year in the United States approximately one half of one percent (.5%) of the population is diagnosed with some form of Cancer. Most of us have been affected personally by this terrible disease, and we know what a dramatic impact it can have on not only the individual but the family members who are caught up in the worry and stress. Individuals, and their immediate family members, may be so distracted with surviving and coping that dental care is on the bottom of their list of priorities.

Patients lose jobs

From January 2003 through December 2005 (three years), 3.8 million workers were displaced from jobs they had held for at least 3 years. An additional 4.3 million persons were displaced from jobs they had held for less than 3 years, for a combined total of 8.1 million from 2003-2005. On an annual basis the total was 2.7 million, or approximately 1% of the population. After factoring in children and spouses, approximately 2.5 percent of the population was affected by job loss in those years. Financial hardship, changes in dental insurance and shifting health-care priorities were all affected.

Patients change jobs

According to human resources experts working for Monster.com, "Nearly three-in-ten workers plan to look for new job opportunities in 2006 and 41 percent of the group plan to leave their companies by the end of 2007." Such change has obvious impact on patient status in the form of moving, income change, insurance change, schedule change and all of the other events that are part of a patient changing their place of work.

Patients lose insurance

As of 2005, only 55% of Americans under age 65 had dental insurance (mostly through their employers), according to the National Association of Dental Plans. Pressured by the soaring cost of health care, many companies are being forced to take a hard look at how they spend their limited health-care dollars. Dental insurance tops the list of benefits employers are looking to reduce or completely eliminate. Obviously such information is a cause for concern among dental professionals, especially those who rely heavily on insurance plans for patient flow and patient loyalty.

What does this all mean?

The total number of patients moving out of your county or further (5.8%), combined with patients who die (1%), already totals nearly 7%. With job loss and divorce the total easily exceeds 10%. This does not even begin to factor in all of the other issues that can influence a patient's motivation or ability to go to the dentist such as terminal illness, depression, drug abuse, alcoholism, mental illness, and a score of other issues, none of which can be controlled by great customer service or quality dental care.

As I've stated many times in this chapter, you must have a plan in place to replace the patients who are lost to everyday attrition. Both internal marketing and external marketing tactics must be implemented. And, the goal ought to be much more than just replacing those patients that are lost. The objective should be to always be expanding your patient base. As the saying goes, "If you're not growing, you are dying."

A growing practice is important, but replacing lost patients needs to be the number one priority of your marketing plan. Never underestimate how many patients you actually lose.

CASE
PRESENTATION

"Case presentation" is a fancy way to say sales pitch

Hopefully this bold statement won't cause the readers of this book to think I'm underestimating what goes on in their offices. I know that as dentists you don't like the word "sales" to show up very often, but I'll apologize now before you read too far into this chapter.

> *"Most of the amenities of modern life are ours because of salesmanship. Everything that goes into the building and upkeep of the home and the conduct of modern business is possible because, somewhere in the process, salesmanship has played its part."*
>
> *– Percy W. Ward in Make Selling Your Career*

The world's economy is driven by the ability of individuals to sell products and services at a profit to other individuals–then reinvesting the profits back into the market as they become buyers of some other product or service. Sales, not money, makes the world go around.

In his massive Handbook on marketing, Dr. Paul H. Nystrom draws a distinction between "selling" and "salesmanship." "Salesmanship is the skill or art of presentation of goods so as to convert neutral or even negative attitudes towards them into positive wants or demand. Salesmanship," he continues, "is the plus factor in selling that induces more transactions and produces more sales than would otherwise occur."

Although subtle selling should happen at many times during a patient's visit, the moment of case presentation is where the serious selling needs to happen. Because this moment is critical, and because so many practices fail to make this brief moment really count, I've dedicated the largest chapter in this book to case presentation. Following these basic but powerful selling concepts will bring a new level of success and fun to your world of dentistry.

Learn the art of selling and your practice will flourish. And you'll have a lot of fun doing it.

Qualities of every great salesperson

In addition to knowing the features and benefits of his or her product, the salesperson of goods or services is faced with the problem of learning how to sell in such a way that the prospect will *want* to buy.

The moral qualities needed in selling dentistry or any other product are the qualities of any good citizen. These qualities are simply and completely covered by the Golden Rule.

A dentist that understands sales knows that he or she will be very unhappy, if treatment is sold that the patient doesn't really need or may not be happy with. Such a dentist knows that peace of mind and long-term reputation, require strong, positive, personal qualities.

Honesty is a must. It gives case presentation a sincere quality, and creates a bond of sympathy between patient and dentist and usually it changes a patient's lack of interest. Patients will always prefer to be treated by a dentist who is sincerely enthusiastic about his or her services and craft, and the dentist's sincerity gives the patient confidence in both the service and the practice.

If all else fails, treat people like you'd like to be treated.

The fake smile

A fake smile will never be a substitute for personality. The smile a patient is greeted with needs to be based on the skills and the service the dentist is willing to provide. Confidence, integrity, and a feeling of happiness are emotions the patient will see as authentic.

Great case presentation requires study as well as experience. Ambitious salesmen read widely, not only in business and technical literature, but in everyday subjects–business, philosophy, sports and current events. It will always pay to be well spoken in areas of interest which patients enjoy discussing.

An old saying I learned years ago, has always helped me understand the art of understanding sales prospects. It goes like this:

"If you can see the world through Jim Jones' eyes, you can sell Jim Jones what Jim Jones buys."

Really listen to your patients

One skill of great case presentation is listening for what the patient is really saying. The basketball player might say, "Yeah, I can hit that foul shot," but he might say it with his eyes cast down. Great dental salespeople have to have a tremendous capacity for focusing on what's really bothering the patient, so they can make the right decision for both the patient and the practice. Dentists who do all the talking during a case presentation not only bore the patient, but also generally lose the sale. You should be listening at least 50 percent of the time. You can improve your listening skills by taking notes, observing your patient's body language, not jumping to conclusions, and concentrating on what your patient is really saying.

Remember: body language makes up 55% of all communication. The tone and pace of a patient's communication makes up 38% of their communication and finally, words make up only 7% of a patient's communication.

Don't get fooled... Understanding how a patient <u>really</u> feels can be tricky.

Focus on the second sale

Studies show that nearly a high percentage of all dental sales are produced by word of mouth. They're the result of a patient telling a friend, family member or associate to buy a product or service because the patient was satisfied. With that data in mind, every time you provide treatment your whole dental team must concentrate on developing future and referral business with each patient. Every move you make must be aimed at the second sale. Ask yourself: Will this be such a great experience that my patient will make me a life-long care provider and always feel comfortable referring friends and family?

Never "live for the moment" when it comes to winning patients.

Ask questions carefully

Ask questions that require more than a "yes" or "no" answer, and questions that deal with more than just price and the technical aspects of the dental treatment. Most importantly, ask questions that will reveal your patient's motivation to purchase, their problems and needs, and their decision-making processes. Don't be afraid to ask a patient why he or she feels a certain way, That's how you'll learn to understand your patients and ultimately help them accept treatment that's best for them.

Talk 20% of the time and listen 80%. You'll be amazed at what you hear.

Keep probing

If a patient tells you, "I'm just trying to do what's most affordable right now," do you immediately tell him how your diagnosis is the most affordable way to take care of their dental problem? A smart treatment presenter won't. He or she will ask more questions and keep probing for the real issue. For example: "I understand why that is important. Can you tell me more about your concern"? Ask for as much information as possible so you can better position your treatment plan and show that you understand your patient's needs.

Dig, Dig, Dig.

Write down objections

Show your patient you are carefully listening
to what they are saying by writing down their
objections. When a patient notices that you are actually
documenting their concerns they will be more careful
to give detailed answers that are accurate with their
feelings. This method of communication will also help
you specifically answer their objections by showing how
they will benefit from your treatment plan. It could be,
for instance, a scheduling issue or that they are really
just afraid of the potential pain from the procedure.
Sometimes just giving your patient more than one option
will help you identify their true objection instead of a
generic excuse.

Get out a pen and write while you listen.

Turn a negative into a positive

If you are a recently graduated dentist and haven't sold
a particular treatment before, don't worry. You can
phrase your case presentation like this: "Not one patient
in a thousand has ever experienced the advantages of this
new implant system or this new same day crown." It really
is very simple, and the typical patient will never know this

may be the first time you've ever sold a full orthodontic case or prepped teeth for a new metal-free bridge.

Make being new a good thing.

Offer a worry-free guarantee

Let your patients know their satisfaction is guaranteed. A simple and easy-to-understand guarantee minimizes customer objections and shows that you believe in your dental services. A good guarantee should be unconditional and should not include hidden clauses, like "guaranteed for only 6 months." As a dental service provider, a good phrase to use is "Your Satisfaction Guaranteed." You'll be thrilled with our service or we'll redo it at our expense.

The cost of any re-do's will more than make up for the increased case acceptance you'll experience.

Change your vocabulary

Patients hate medical terminology. Especially when it sounds scary and expensive. You won't impress your patients by speaking "over their heads." Humanize the way you tell them they have a chronic skin disease called atopic dermatitis or that there are indications of non-carious cervical lesions.

Remember how you felt your first day in dental school when you're tempted to use scientific lingo.

Sell benefits, not features

The biggest mistake dentists make in case presentation is focusing on what their proposed treatment *is*. Rather, it's how it will make the patient feel that's important. A dental implant is a titanium post that is placed in the jawbone to permanently replace a missing tooth or teeth. That's what it *is*. What the implant *does* is make your patients smile more, look younger, feel more confident in social situations. Always concentrate on how your dental services will benefit your patient.

A story is told on this point by Robert E. Moore in his book published last year: The Human Side of Selling. A salesman was trying to sell a stove to an elderly lady. He described the construction features at great length, talked about B.T.U.s, thermostats and automatic damper control. Then the customer interrupted him with this wonderfully human question: "Tell me, mister, will it keep an old lady warm?"

Focus on how treatment will benefit the patient. Don't worry so much about how it does it.

Differentiate your product

Why should a patient accept treatment from you and not from another dentist? I suggest coming up with at least three benefits that will give a customer a reason to accept your treatment plan. Many patients don't like to go out of their comfort zone to try something new. So, give them three good reasons to say yes. Your dental services or dental product should look better, be a better value, and made of better materials.

Make your product unique and special to every patient.

Offer two choices

Instead of just asking, "How does this sound?"–give your patient a choice. For example, when proposing a three unit posterior bridge, ask them if they would rather have a traditional PFM bridge or a newer, but slightly more expensive, metal-free bridge. When they state their choice, schedule the appointment for the bridge prep. The patient is not likely to stop you, because emotionally they realize they've committed and they've said 'yes.'

Ask patients to choose option "a" or option "b" It's simple, but it works.

It's not a veneer, it's a "Brand X" veneer

One of the most under-utilized selling concepts for great case presentation, is that of positioning your services along with the brands and materials associated with the treatment. For example, I teach dentists to never propose only generic veneers as part of a their treatment plan. Always explain to the patient that you will be placing "Brand X" veneers or "Brand Y" or whatever system you prefer. As a dentist, you've picked that system over the others for a good reason. Make sure you tell the patient why. It will add real depth and sizzle to your case presentation. This strategy should be used with every important system you provide such as, implants, inlays, crowns, bridges, whitening and on and on and on.

Attach your case presentation to brand names. It will ad an important level of credibility.

Answer objections with "feel, felt, found"

Don't lose your enthusiasm for the presentation when a patient says, "I'm not interested," "It's too expensive," or "I don't have time right now." Simply say, "I understand how you _**feel**_. A lot of my patients have _**felt**_ the same way. But when they _**found**_ out how much better their smile looked, they were amazed." Then ask them if they are sure about their decision. They've usually changed their minds. This is a trick that effective salespeople have used for years to respond to objections.

Try it... It really works.

A picture says it all

We live in an incredibly visual society. 3-D animation that "looks so real you could almost touch it," is everywhere. Giant television screens with high resolution displays are in millions of homes. Video game are more realistic every year. And, color printers can be purchased for a lot less than $100. As the saying goes, "a picture is worth a thousand words." Make absolutely sure that you are using high quality visual aids in every part of case presentation.

Stop sketching illustrations with a ball-point pen and stop using the plastic models you've had since dental school. Your patients deserve better.

Use technology

Dentists now have access to many powerful case presentation tools that are delivered on DVD, over the internet or through interactive software programs. The days of charts and posters on the wall are gone. Drawing a picture of a root canal on a yellow pad of lined paper are especially gone. Implement technology as part of your case presentation. Your patients will never see your practice the same again.

3-D animation on a flat-screen display or a plastic tooth model you've used since dental school. It's up to you.

Send home a treatment plan

When you visit a car dealer to look at a new Lexus, you usually go home with a sexy, full-color brochure that almost smells like a new car. Car dealers do this because it works. My company has developed a powerful, and easy-to-use treatment plan builder, that lets you send every patient home with a full-color proposal. It has shown to improve case acceptance dramatically. It protects you from cancellations and it is a strong part of the overall brand-building experience.

Check it out at www.idmtools.com

TECHNOLOGY

Hey! It's the 21ˢᵗ Century

As of the writing of this book, personal computers have been around for a good twenty years now. The Internet has been available everywhere for at least ten years. Color printers cost less than a hundred dollars. And, dental practice management software was available before 1990. With that being said, why in the **?#@%!** do I still find that dentists don't even own a modern computer. Too many don't even have access to the Internet in their offices. What gives? If you want to build a brand, attract sophisticated patients, retain employees and obtain patient referrals, and you don't utilize technology everywhere, the odds are stacked against you.

Go digital now! Before it is too late to catch up.

High speed internet

The Internet is amazing. The amount of information that you can obtain in seconds is almost impossible to describe. Clinical training, online purchasing, dental forums, dental news, pharmaceutical information, e-mail, rapid insurance claim processing, online file storage, and patient education systems, all require Internet access. Anything but high-speed access is too cumbersome to deal with. And, it's very affordable. I've heard excuses like, "I'm afraid that my staff will waste time surfing the internet," or "I've done fine up until now without it." Or, "I missed that whole computer thing while I was in dental school." I don't buy it. And neither should you. It's kind of like the memo that circulated through the management team at IBM in the 1970's that said, "Why would anyone want to own their own computer?"

Not having high speed Internet in your office in the 21st century, would have been like riding a horse to your practice in 1965.

A computer in every operatory

The age of chairside scheduling, and charting is here. In fact, it has been here for a while now. Accessing photos, video clips, DVDs, digital x-rays and on and on will not only make you more efficient but will send a message to your patients that you are all about the best care. Your patients may not be able to examine your crown preps or your artistry inside a root canal, but they do notice technology. Many of your patients notice technology because they work with it professionally. If for no other reason, make the investment to chairside computers to enhance your case presentation skills. You'll be surprised by how quickly the investment will pay for itself.

Computers must be a priority in any practice.

DVD Players

A good DVD player is now less than $100. I don't know how they do it, but I'm not asking any questions. Flat panel televisions and computer displays have also plummeted in price. For operatories, I often recommend the portable DVD players that can be given to the patient to hold in their lap. It makes such a great impression and they can be purchased for a few hundred dollars. There are a lot of great resources available to dentists for case presentation and patient education, make sure you take advantage of everything you can get your hands on.

Be able to play DVDs in every treatment room and in your reception area.

Color Printers

Like all electronic equipment, color printers have become amazingly affordable. They used to cost big bucks are were a pain to maintain. Today, a color printer costs so little, that they have become an almost disposable item. Not only are they cheap to operate but the quality is amazing. In fact, it's good enough that photo developing labs have lost a huge chunk of market share to consumers who now print their own photos at home. While reading this book, you'll hear me explain several times how important it is to send patients home with a printed treatment plan. These documents must be in color to have any impact on the patient. Digital imaging and pre-op photography are just two more reasons to have at least one good color computer on hand in your office. Ink-jet printers are great for photos and color laser printers can print a document in just a few seconds. Do your research and get the model that best fits your needs.

Consumers love color. Don't be a black and white dentist any longer.

Digital imaging and radiography

The future of dentistry is extremely bright. The technology around the corner will completely change the way dental procedures are delivered to patients. However, don't wait for tomorrow. The products and technology already on the market offer some amazing advancements that you can have today. Among these advancements are digital radiography and its twin sister, digital imaging. My partner is a practicing general dentist in Salt Lake City, Utah. His name is

Dr. Robert Thorup and he was one of the first dentists in the country to implement digital radiography in a dental practice. Digital imaging soon followed. Dr. Rob lectures nationally on digital imaging and radiography and how to implement both technologies into the everyday practice. Whenever I listen to him speak, I'm in awe of the technology and how affordable it is when viewed from a business perspective. What impresses me the most, is being able to visually show a patient their particular diagnosis. This is a powerful marketing tactic and critical to great case presentation.

Rob's opinion is that digital radiography saves time and money (more than most dentists really understand), and the Holy Grail of this technology is digital intra-oral imaging. Color images do several things: they increase patient knowledge about needed treatment, they cause patients to act on needed treatment, and they give legal proof of needed treatment (just to name a few). If you get the opportunity to view this technology in action, whether through a lecture or a CE course, you'll be amazed.

Digital Radiography and Imaging are here to stay. What are you waiting for?

Know your materials

Remember that dental materials class you had in dental school? Here is where it will pay off. Are all composites created equal? Are all crowns created equal? Absolutely not. Most practices still offer silver and tooth colored filling materials. But what kind of composite material are they placing in the patient's mouth? Hybrid or Micro-hybrid? Layered or just "thumb printed" in the prep?

At the time of this writing the least expensive hybrid composite is about $9.30 per gram. The most expensive micro hybrid composite is more than double the cost at $20.03 per gram. As of today, a dentist can purchase a basic crown for around $100, or he or she can purchase a multi layered, internally and externally stained crown for about $285. That's not to mention all of the different types and brands of crowns that are out there. Whitening agents also have similar ranges in cost and quality.

Now for the million dollar question; how can one CDT code cover all of the porcelain and PFM crown types in modern dentistry? It can't! If you know and understand modern materials, and know when and where to use them, you can turn this wide variety of materials into into an effective treatment and business tool within your dental practice. I know a Dentist in California who absolutely loves a particular type and brand of crown. A lab in Texas charges him $265 per unit. That is $130 more that he normally pays for an all porcelain crown from the lab down the street. He charges patients who chooses to upgrade, an additional $260 for this specific crown. His philosophy is this: "There isn't a business in the country that doesn't mark up value-added products and services."

Learn your materials, and learn to use them to empower your patients and to the benefit of your business.

COSMETIC FANTASY LAND

I know a dentist in Florida...

About a year ago I worked with a dentist in an exclusive area of California. I'll call him Dr. Anderson for the purposes of this story. He was convinced that he was going to be the next great thing in cosmetic dentistry. He believed that he had everything he needed—advanced training, the right location, the right dental team and on and on.

Dr. Anderson was personal friends with another dentist who had "made it big," and his friend was in the process of developing a television show that would be aired all over Florida. He went on to tell me that the money was flowing for his dentist friend and that he was getting upwards of $50,000 for a full-mouth case. The secret to his friend's success was a very expensive advertising campaign. He was running ads everywhere, and was going to show Dr. Anderson how it was done. In fact, he convinced Dr. Anderson to "sign up" with the same advertising agency that had helped the friend in Florida get rich.

After doing my best to "stop the runaway train", I finally bowed-out and let him retain this hot ad agency that had fully convinced him that a lifestyle of fame and fortune was his for the taking. He spent almost $100,000 in radio, television, giant billboards and a local Extreme

Makeover type television show with the local news channel in California.

After this entire whirlwind of advertising, the dentist had received twenty one new patients. Only a few of them were interested in full-mouth restorations, and of those, only one accepted the treatment plan for the pricey procedure. The others who accepted treatment were more interested in a few anterior crowns or whitening. From these patients, Dr. Anderson was able to retain a few of them as regular patients, and did a fair amount of restorative dentistry.

The revenue total for all of this dentistry left Dr. Anderson with a loss of about $35,000. And, that was stretching it. In fact, the full mouth case that he performed ended up being a very difficult case with a very picky patient. The re-makes and adjustments probably ate up more profit than Dr. Anderson was willing to admit.

There are a lot of reasons this "extreme marketing" effort failed. Many of them are described in this book. Too much reach and not enough frequency was a major mistake. No offer, a confusing message, poor case presentation and not understanding personality profiles are just a few of the others.

If it sounds too good to be true, it probably is.

Cosmetic Fantasy Land

The biggest mistake was positioning. Or, in other words, Dr. Anderson picked the wrong product to promote. It is very difficult to create a marketing strategy around cosmetic dentistry that actually "pulls" well enough to have an acceptable return on investment. At our company we call this "Cosmetic Fantasy Land." I'm not saying that big cosmetic cases aren't out there. What I am saying is that it is financially foolish to create a one-dimensional marketing plan, and bet the farm on that plan, without knowing more about what results to expect.

All over the country there are dental seminars, institutes of higher learning and experts that evangelize huge professional and financial gains from focusing solely on cosmetic cases. Be wary of these messages. They can be misleading and frequently exaggerate the benefits of targeting just cosmetic dentistry.

In my experience with hundreds of practices from all over the country, I have never come across a practice that is consistently selling enough big cases to pay all the bills, let alone thrive. It's mostly big talk and posturing by the practice, when in reality, most of their profit is being generated by everyday, meat-and-potatoes restorative dentistry. Of course, there are exceptions to the rule, but the examples are few and far between.

Believe it when you see it. Until then, don't.

Look within your own practice

The important observation to make is that most cosmetic dentistry is not sold through advertising campaigns and new patient acquisition tactics. Most cosmetic procedures are performed on patients who are already patients of record. Some of them see the same dentist for years before considering cosmetic procedures. One of the problems I see, is that it may be years before these patients are educated by the practice on what cosmetic options are available. Nearly every dentist who is looking for an increase in cosmetic and implant cases, will benefit dramatically by doing a better job of education and case presentation within his or her own patient-base.

Another important observation some dentists have already made is this: Patients who can afford cosmetic dentistry usually already have a dentist. Or, they have a friend or family member they will go to for a referral. Cosmetic dentistry, for the most part, is expensive. And, because we live in a social food chain, those who want it know how to get it, and rarely make an appointment with an unknown dentist just because they saw a magazine ad.

Your best cosmetic candidate already has a file and may be in your chair today.

Open your own mouth

I won't go into too much detail here, because I've dedicated a whole chapter to case presentation that you may have already read. However, don't forget that selling cosmetic dental procedures requires a sales process. That process includes great verbal communication skills and ever-improving case presentation. I know that asking your patients to open their mouths is a daily part of your life, but maybe you should consider how effective you are when you open your own mouth.

Read the chapter on case presentation. Then read it again.

PERSONALITY PROFILES AND MARKETING

Personalities in Dentistry

I know a dentist that was having a very difficult time getting a long time denture wearer to consider a dental implant procedure. Her patient seemed perfectly happy to talk about his family or his latest vacation. But when this young dentist tried to talk implants, the patient clammed up every time.

Then Dr. Jones (I'll call her that) realized she was dealing with a different personality type. So, over time on subsequent visits she changed her approach and started working with the patient in a much softer kind of approach.

During a follow-up appointment, she spent several minutes talking with him about the car he was restoring and his son who played football for a local college. With about 10 minutes of the appointment left, the patient started to explain he was having problems with his dentures and asked Dr. Jones if she could help. She said, "I think we can help. I'll consider the best approach. What do you say we get back together next week?" She already had the answer, but her patient didn't want the answer right away. He wanted to get back together the next week and talk about it. "I can't even total the amount of dentistry we sold him over the next couple of years," Dr. Jones says.

Dr. Jones' success shows how important it is for

dental teams to recognize and adjust to the different personalities that walk through their practice. The more comfortable a dental team can make a patient feel, the more likely he or she is to accept treatment. I'd even go so far to say, that it's more important that the patient likes or respects you than they like your dental products or services.

Your patients buy things from people they like, respect and trust. They buy from people who seem to be like themselves. "It is our job to become the emotional equal of our prospect," says sales consultant and sales veteran Ray Leone.

What the experts say

In his sales training courses, the president of Leone Resource Group in Charleston, S.C., devotes half the time allotted just to building rapport and understanding personalities, with the rest devoted to product presentation. "If you don't have rapport, which generates trust and having that client open up to you and breaking down all the barriers of communication, there's no point in going forward," he says.

A crucial part of developing rapport is understanding the type of personalities you encounter. After correctly assessing the client's personality, the salesperson can better predict what kind of person the client trusts and what kind of information he or she will want.

Assessing a new patient's personality can even help you determine at the very beginning of the presentation whether or not to try for the first-appointment close. Patients process information differently and go at different rates of speed. If you are dealing with an engineer or somebody who writes code for Microsoft, that's not the same as if you're presenting to a marketing specialist like me, who likes the big picture.

Patients are so diverse in the way they process information and the amount of information they want. You must adjust your entire case presentation almost from "Hello," because each patient requires totally different opens, middles and closes.

Basics of D.I.S.C.

Fortunately, there's a guide to help sales professionals figure out which personality type they're dealing with. In the early 1920's, American psychologist William Moulton Marston created a system for categorizing personality types, which many salespeople now use to help them better understand their clients. Inspired by findings from Swiss psychologist Carl Jung, the system contains four personality types represented in the acronym DISC. Different people give different names to each letter, but the same four personalities are represented: dominant (also called driver), interpersonal (or interactive), security-minded (or steadfast), and critical thinker (also called cautious).

No one falls purely within any of these categories. But you can observe your patients to see which characteristic is most prominent. And don't forget to make a note of it in their chart.

Each personality type has different interests, motivations and fears. So they have different criteria for accepting treatment. The D (dominant) must respect you to buy from you; the I (interpersonal) must like you; the S (security-minded) must trust you; and with the C (critical thinker) you don't even enter into the decision. All you have to do is provide them with the data.

Some patients are more likely to "move-away" while others "move-forward." With the analytical and safety-minded patient, you may not want to be in a rush to thrust your hand out to shake it. S-types want their private space and before they'll shake your hand, they may want to get more comfortable with you. However, the driver will walk into your office, grab your hand and say, "I need a crown."

Dominants and Interpersonals are generally impatient people. Dominants especially want to move quickly and make it happen. D's and I's will accept treatment right on the spot.

S's and C's rarely accept treatment during the first visit. This doesn't mean these patients won't want you to give them all the information. They just need time. If you go through a complete treatment presentation, including pricing and closing at the end, they may call back and schedule treatment after they've had a chance to digest the information. If you go for a close on the spot with a C, you've messed up big-time.

Once you've determined which half of the DISC a client falls on, you can narrow it down to the exact type by asking one question, depending on which side they fall on.

If they're outgoing, you say, "Is this person more of a relater of people or a director of people?" If you believe they're a director of people, then they're a D. If you think they're a relater, then they're an I.

If they're reserved, you ask yourself another question: Is this person more accepting of people or assessing? Acceptors are S's, assessors are C's.

Here's a more detailed look at each personality type and how to approach them:

Personality types defined

D Personalities–This style represents 18-20 percent of all people.

D's are doers. Some refer to them as drivers because they're the people who make things happen. Business owners and doctors often fall into this category. They're dominant, high-risk takers and, as a result, quite often end up at the top of an organization. As the name implies, drivers want things to move quickly. A highly dominant person is going to be very much a bottom-line patient. They'll tell you this is what they want and they don't want to hear a lot of fluff because they don't have time for that conversation.

I Personalities–This style represents 28 percent of all people.

As the label suggests, I's make relationships a top priority. They want to spend their time talking to the dentist. They're concerned about who's going to be working on their teeth and what their neighbors and friends think. So in discussion of the choices they need to make, high-I clients will ask what other people like and what most people do. They want to stand out in a crowd, so they want the best-looking smile available. Their primary fear is social acceptance. I's also like the most cutting-edge gadgets, partially because of their love for life and partly because of the prestige. They tend to be very enthusiastic, and they hate detail. You may not want to go through the detail of an implant system, they may just want to see a lot of color pictures and 3-D animation.

S Personalities–This is where 40 percent of people are found.

S's hate disruption, hassle, change and risk. They sometimes drive Volvos. They're very safety-minded, they want side-impact airbags and two seat belts instead of one. They want to check the product thoroughly– that's how they make a decision. They'll look at all the ingredients on a cereal box to make sure they're comfortable with it. These personalities gravitate toward professions such as nursing, teaching and jobs that require teamwork. They like to work in teams, are very family-oriented, resist sudden changes and take longer to do things than D's or I's.

You may find these patients the most challenging because their cautious nature keeps them from getting too enthusiastic about anything. They tend to be factually driven. They don't get emotional one way or the other. When working with these clients, give them a lot of information and don't pressure them to make a decision. "You just need to give them a lot more time," he says. Also, be extra careful about keeping appointments and staying on schedule with these patients.

C Personalities–This style represents only 14 percent of the population.

Critical thinkers are very similar to security-minded patients, except that they take more enjoyment from technical information and analyzing the situation before accepting treatment. These patients will often work with numbers and technology. They are usually engineers, computer specialists, chief financial officers, purchasing managers, code writers, quality control inspectors and accountants. You can identify them because they're asking questions about everything. This behavior is motivated by the C's greatest fear of making a mistake –any kind of mistake. They figure the more time they take to analyze, the less chance they have of being wrong. That's why you'll never get a C to accept treatment on the spot. Like S's, these patients require more time to make decisions. Like S's, these clients aren't crazy about risk. So the most cutting-edge products don't usually appeal to them. "To the high-I, innovation means new and first and that's what they want," Leone says. "To a high-C, new means untested."

Learn how to deal with different personalities and you'll unlock one of the best-kept secrets to marketing success.

GROW, PROFIT, THRIVE.

A CASE STUDY

This case study is real. However, to maintain anonymity, the names have been changed to protect the innocent. (Is that from Dragnet?)

Case Study: Dr. Nelson
Pre-Marketing Facts

Practice Name: Perry S. Nelson D.D.S.

Practice location: The practice is located in Phoenix, Arizona. The office is one unit of a four-plex of medical offices. The other offices are occupied by a Family Physician, an Orthodontist and an Optometrist. The office is on a major street near downtown Phoenix. Parking is somewhat limited and the signage is nonexistent other than a small brick marquis.

Overview of the facility: The practice is approximately fifteen years old, as is most of the dental equipment and furnishings. The office has a modest reception area, one hygiene room and two operatories. The practice does not use digital radiography. Dentrix is utilized in the front office only, and has not been updated for a few years. Internet connection is in the dentist's personal office and is not high-speed. The two computers in the practice are fairly outdated. The office has no color printer. The office has no DVD players, only a VHS player in the reception area for kids movies.

Services provided: Dr. Nelson provides basic restorative dental services as well as limited cosmetics. All large cases as well as implants are referred to specialists. All root canal therapy is also referred out. Periodontal therapy is significant and creates a healthy percentage of monthly revenue. Many of the patients are low-income and require PPO participation. Dr. Nelson utilizes a local crown and bridge lab with very little cosmetic experience. The relationship has existed for nearly a decade. The lab is consistent and creates great fitting basic crowns, but offers only one type of metal-free restoration which is too weak for posteriors or bridges.

Patient count: Over 1,500 patient files, however production does not reflect such a practice size. It is likely that many of the patients are visiting other dentists or that recall efforts are weak.

Team structure: One full-time dentist (Dr. Nelson), one hygienist, two assistants and an office manager.

Days worked: Monday through Thursday, 8:00-5:00 with a one hour break for lunch. Telephone answering machine is turned on during lunch and on Friday.

New patient flow: New patient flow is not tracked accurately, but seems to be approximately 8-10 per month. Summertime is slowest.

Monthly production: Average monthly production is $55,000. Receivables typically exceed $100,000.

The Story

Our company was contacted by Dr. Nelson after he attended a marketing seminar we held Phoenix, Arizona. He was finding it difficult to maintain consistency in new patient flow and was concerned that his practice was becoming more and more controlled by PPO plans. He was interested in providing more cosmetic and implant dentistry but was concerned that his facility and image would be an obstacle. He was also experiencing cash-flow problems and was concerned that his front-office team needed more operational training. Dr. Nelson was comfortable that his assistants and hygienist were capable of new change and worked well together as a team. Case presentation was non-existent other than basic discussion of diagnosis with patients.

After several lengthy discussions with a marketing consultant in our company, a very detailed marketing plan was outlined and approved by Dr. Nelson. The plan was to be initially implemented over a twelve month period, after which a second plan would be created for subsequent years. Dr. Nelson was prepared to make a sizeable investment in the plan as well as an investment in upgraded equipment and technology systems. He was excited and at the same time nervous. He had never done any practice marketing and was hoping to make some dramatic changes in the practice.

Dr. Nelson had purchased the practice from another dentist after working as his associate for two years. Although his mentor was a very wonderful person, his old-school mentality and bad habits rubbed off on Dr. Nelson to the point, that he was in a real rut when we met. What he needed was his own "Extreme Makeover."

It was determined that Dr. Nelson needed to make a few basic technology equipment purchases so that he could properly implement the proposed plan. High speed internet access was brought into the practice and made available in every room including the treatment rooms.

Dr. Nelson worked with his practice management software provider to upgrade to the latest version, which gave him chair-side scheduling and access to patient records. Dr. Nelson also purchased new computers with large flat screens and the ability to play DVDs. These computers were placed so that patients were able to view the screen. Each computer was networked to a color laser printer. The reception area was also outfitted with a large plasma screen, professionally mounted to the wall, and connected to a DVD player at the front desk.

Due to budget restraints, Dr. Nelson decided to wait several months to implement digital radiography. His plan was to also replace his chairs and delivery systems at the same time. The priority early in the plan was new patient flow and case acceptance. The new equipment would have to wait for a while.

Although the marketing plan created for Dr. Nelson was much more detailed, here is a summary of the proposal.

The Strategy

A. Triple the new patient flow. At least one new patient everyday was the initial goal.

B. Dramatically improve case presentation and case acceptance.

C. Create a fresh, new brand image.

D. Dramatically improve patient referrals.

E. Improve profitability

The Tactics

New name and practice identity: As mentioned already in this book, changing a practice name after years of familiarity can be a tricky thing. However, it was determined that Dr. Nelson's name would still appear as the main header and the new practice name would be a subtitle to his name. Over two or three years, the new name would replace Dr. Nelson's but it would be done very carefully. After a creative development process was complete, a new logo was finished and new practice name created. This new identity would be used everywhere. Among other things, new window signs, letterhead, envelopes, appointment cards and patient forms were created with a fresh new look and feel that became the beginning of a new brand for Dr. Nelson.

Internet Site: As a component of the new name and image, a powerful new internet site was quickly developed. This site was deep in dental content and educational information. In addition to standard HTML, the content was published using: video clips, Flash animation, detailed illustrations and 3-D graphics. The site also contained frequently asked dental questions, insurance information, overviews of the dental team and the ability to request an appointment. The Internet address was prominently promoted on every marketing component to make patients very aware of the new site.

Referral Brochure: To better enable the process of receiving referrals from existing patients, a referral brochure was designed and sent home with every patient, everyday. This brochure contained an overview of the practice, and when folded, was small enough to fit in a patient's pocket or purse. Three thousand copies were printed as a one year supply.

Direct Mail: One of the main strategies for Dr. Nelson's marketing plan was to increase patient flow. In fact, it was probably the most important part of the overall plan. A detailed demographic study of the area surrounding

Dr. Nelson's practice became the foundation for the mail campaign. A large, oversized, postcard was designed. The postcard was full-color on both sides, and utilized beautiful photography and graphic design. The quantity of direct mail determined to be most appropriate for Dr. Nelson's goals was 5,000 postcards sent monthly. The mailing lists purchased had 15,000 homes matching the targeted demographics as well as all new move-ins in the area. Each homeowner would receive a postcard four times per year. The postcard also included several time-sensitive offers to create a sense of urgency for individuals who received the mail pieces. The internet site was displayed prominently on the card with another special available for individuals who visited the website.

Local Business Flyer: Another effective external marketing component was the development of a flyer that was placed in the offices of local businesses, such as: fitness centers, cosmetic surgeons, and family physicians. Each flyer contained the same offers as the direct mail postcard. The flyer was displayed in an attractive acrylic stand. 1,500 flyers were printed for the first year.

Patient Rewards: Dr. Nelson's office manager was trained to utilize a new system designed by our company that makes it easy to send a gift to a patient who has referred a friend or family member. The system is called

"Patient Rewards" and gave Dr. Nelson's office the ability to quickly generate a thank-you card and purchase a gift such as, Mrs. Field's Cookies. Sending professional gift packages to patients who refer has been shown to be a very powerful internal marketing tool and the Patient Rewards system makes it convenient and easy.

Wall Art: Dr. Nelson was provided with ten, large-format, pieces of wall art that portrayed a variety of individuals with great healthy smiles. This wall art was customized for Dr. Nelson's office and each piece included his logo and marketing message. For example, one of the pieces was of a beautiful woman in her late thirties with a gorgeous smile. The customized message was, "Ask Dr. Nelson how to remake your smile with Brand X Veneers." Each piece was framed to match his new paint and interior colors.

Patient Survey: To obtain as much information as possible about Dr. Nelson's existing patient base, a series of quarterly patient surveys were sent to all patients of record. The surveys were delivered with postage already paid to facilitate responses. Each survey asked for feedback in customer experience and requested response to several key areas of interest. These surveys have shown to be a critical form of data gathering to best determine where a practice is succeeding or needs to improve. The surveys can be returned anonymously or with a name.

Patient Letters: A quarterly letter was also written on Dr. Nelson's behalf and sent to patients of record with the patient surveys already mentioned. The letters were short but informative and always discussed an important dental topic or gave an overview of any new services or technology Dr. Nelson had invested in. The goal was to stay in-touch with each patient and emphasize Dr. Nelson's commitment to provide the best care possible.

On-Hold Message: An on-hold messaging device with a professionally recorded audio track was implemented with Dr. Nelson's phone system. The looping audio segment included brief overviews of new services and technology available at Dr. Nelson's practice, as well as a reminder of special offers for new patients. The audio file was ten minutes in length and automatically looped when attached to the phone system.

Treatment PRO: To ensure that case presentation was perfected, Treatment PRO was implemented in Dr. Nelson's practice. This system was developed by our company and includes four key modules that make case presentation and patient education extremely effective in a short period of time. The system includes a Reception Area DVD, Operatory DVD, Treatment Plan Booklet and software that easily creates beautiful Treatment Plans to send home with patients. Dr. Nelson's entire team was trained to use the system and operating policies were put in place to standardize each team member's presentation.

After 30 Days

During the first 30 days the logo and all associated identity components were completed. Treatment PRO was implemented and all training completed. The Internet site was completed. The direct mail postcard was designed and printed, including the demographic study. The on-hold messaging system was completed and installed. Dr. Nelson's team reported a substantial improvement in case acceptance due to Treatment PRO. Many patients began to compliment the practice on their new image and how impressive it seemed to be.

After 90 Days

All other components outlined in the proposal were delivered within the first 60 days. Within 90 days two mailings of 5,000 pieces had been mailed. New patient flow was exceeding 30 new patients monthly.

After 12 Months

At the completion of the campaign, Dr. Nelson had obtained over 300 new patients. Case acceptance sky-rocketed due to Treatment PRO and an overhaul of the practice's product offerings. Patients were referring more than ever before. Many new fee-for-service patients were added, while other existing patients adjusted to the new fees and payment policies. At the end of the 12 month marketing program, Dr. Nelson was assisted with a marketing-maintenance program that was more affordable but continued to reinforce the value of his new and improved brand-image and dental practice.

Post-Marketing Facts

Improvements to the facility: Substantial improvements were made including, new computers, DVD players, upgraded software, and digital imaging. Dr. Nelson also dramatically improved the interior and exterior of the office with paint, carpet, cabinets, signage and wall art. New chairs and delivery systems were also added towards the end of the first year.

Services provided: In addition to basic crowns, bridges and fillings, Dr. Nelson retained the services of a new lab and began to offer several all-porcelain restorative systems. Dr. Nelson also began to utilize almost exclusively, a micro-hybrid composite filling material and raised many of his fees proportionately. Dr. Nelson also took several advanced courses on cosmetic procedures that he had been uncomfortable providing in the past. Treatment PRO gave him and his team an easy approach to promoting these new service profitably.

New patient flow: As previously mentioned, Dr. Nelson was able to obtain aver 300 new patients during his first year as well as displace many "old patients" with new patients who were willing to pay for the best care.

Monthly production: Annual average increased to $82,000 monthly. Receivables were reduced to less than $60,000–a much better ratio when compared to monthly income.

Epilogue

Thank you for reading this book. Hopefully, its contents have opened your eyes to how important effective marketing is for every dental practice. Having your eyes opened is only the beginning. The most important thing you can do now is act on the principles described in this book. Now get going, and make your practice Grow, Profit and Thrive.

About the author

Joel Harris is the co-founder of Intelligent Dental Marketing, the leading marketing company for dental practices. Intelligent Dental Marketing is located in Salt Lake City, Utah and serves the marketing needs of hundreds of dental practices each year. Prior to starting Intelligent Dental Marketing, he was the co-founder of two traditional and digital media agencies that specialized in developing powerful communication tools and systems for large corporations. Some of these companies include: Delta Air Lines, Eastman Kodak, US Steel, Boeing, Samsung, CNN and Time Warner. He lives in Utah.

For speaking engagements or for marketing assistance, Joel Harris can be reached at 877-942-8855 or go to: www.idmtools.com